Unplanned Journey

Matador
9 Priory Business Park,
Wistow Road, Kibworth Beauchamp,
Leicestershire. LE8 0RX
Tel: 0116 279 2299
Email: books@troubador.co.uk
Web: www.troubador.co.uk/matador
Twitter: @matadorbooks

ISBN 978 1784625 115

British Library Cataloguing in Publication Data.
A catalogue record for this book is available from the British Library.

Typeset by Troubador Publishing Ltd, Leicester, UK

Matador is an imprint of Troubador Publishing Ltd

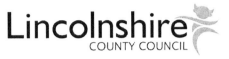

Lincolnshire
COUNTY COUNCIL

discover libraries

This book should be returned on or before the due date.

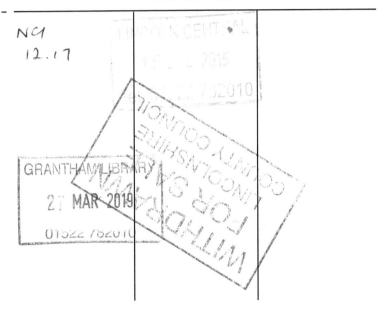
To renew or order library books please telephone 01522 782010
or visit https://lincolnshire.spydus.co.uk
You will require a Personal Identification Number.
Ask any member of staff for this.

The above does not apply to Reader's Group Collection Stock.

Tiggy Walker & Bella West

Unplanned Journey

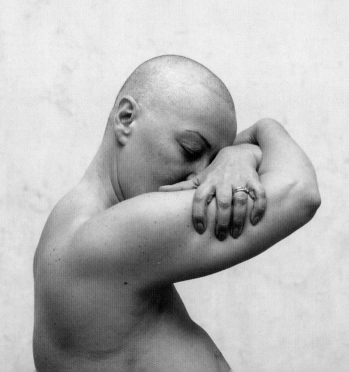

Many people have an unplanned journey.
A journey that is only made bearable by the rock at their side. This book is dedicated to all carers – the selfless givers and unsung heroes who give up their own lives to be that rock.

Tiggy Walker
2015

Before The Journey

November 2013

I am Tiggy Walker. 52 years old. Married. No kids. One dog.

When people meet me the thing they first notice are my large breasts. Some women envy them while occasional men are affected by them. Indeed once I met a retired Admiral at a party who gripped his glass so hard that it shattered spilling red wine all over my cleavage. He apologised saying he was just so excited to meet me. What he meant was 'them'. The sad thing is that I hate 'them'. At 32H they are heavy, get in the way, stop me buying most clothes and only one bra in the country fits. Twice I have met plastic surgeons to discuss a reduction but on moral grounds I decided to keep them. The good Lord made me this way, how could I be so vain etc. etc.

I juggle my time between London, where we have a small flat, and Shaftesbury in Dorset where we are selling our current house, renovating another, and wondering where we shall stay in between the two.

I produce TV commercials. Before marriage I had my own production company. These days I freelance at the wonderful Soho based, Blink. I've made ads for thirty years for everything from bags of salad leaves to flash cars. Right now it's a wax covered Scandinavian cheese.

My husband is Radio 2's Johnnie Walker. Bit of a radio legend, life with him is never dull. Ever. At the epicentre of our lives is his schedule of shows, interviews and other appearances. I am his agent and manager. Indeed I run absolutely every aspect of our busy lives. He is great in the studio. I am rather better at the vast admin of our existence.

In the background I am writing a TV series called "Antonia". This is my passion, yet it gets too little of my time and has yet to flourish.

Finally, I have just agreed to join the Fundraising Board of the charity Carers UK. Having cared for Johnnie when he fought cancer in 2003, I know how tough that role is. I am only too happy to help others who go through similar ordeals.

I used to be incredibly sociable. Right now my perfect evening is spent at home with Johnnie and Darcey the dog in front of the fire watching a couple of episodes of "Breaking Bad".

It's fair to say that I'm struggling to cope. I'm tired, irascible and easily stressed.

But at least we have a great holiday planned. Next month we are off to Australia for three weeks. Starting in Margaret River, we will then take the three day Indian Pacific train journey from Perth to Sydney where my brother Graham lives. He will collect us from Sydney Train Station on Christmas Morning. I can't wait…

12 December 2013

Today is the day of the Blink Christmas lunch and I am sitting in a waiting room, Surgical Outpatients to be precise, at Salisbury District Hospital. Today should have been about celebrating with Blink - I have just produced a particularly stylish cheese commercial for them. It was a fraught, stressful production, but nothing out of the ordinary, nothing compared to what came next. Two weeks ago, whilst the commercial was in post-production, I was showering when I found a lump in my right breast. Two days ago I saw the GP. And in two days time I am off to Australia. I assumed it was a cyst, but to be sure the doc wanted me to get checked out before I left.

I trotted off for my mammogram and ultrasound like an obedient lamb. When the radiographer said he was going to take a biopsy I chirped "What a good idea. As I'm here." It was only when some woman took my hand and looked at me with her kindly yet sad resigned face that I thought, "SHIT. They think it's cancer." Within fifteen minutes I knew that it was. It is not usual to be told at this point. They like the test results back. But I explained I was going away and asked if I could be sent an email. I couldn't. So I was told right then and there.

I cried. I apologised for crying. I drove home crying.

I made an instant decision. I would never produce another commercial. I would also stop managing Johnnie's career.

I stopped in Tollard Royal to walk Darcey the dog. Life had suddenly become heightened. The birdsong was loud and clear, the view towards Win Green beautiful. The dog leaping with joy, it all felt so sharp. For the first time in my life I faced my mortality. There was a strange beauty and calmness to that thought.

I couldn't tell Johnnie. He was doing a reading at a Carol Service for the Pelican Cancer Trust that evening. I couldn't risk him being too upset to take part. I waited till he got home. It was late. "So when will you know?" he asked. "I already do." He took the news very bravely. He was so utterly strong. We clasped on to each other all night long. It seems that only in sickness do we realise how deep the love is.

10 January 2014

We got back from Australia late last night. On just one occasion I shed a few tears. My jaw bone was aching and I thought "Dear God. It's in my bones." Having seen Johnnie almost killed by chemo, and being the organic, nutrient taking, drug hating thing that I am, I have always said I would never have chemo. In the middle of that night I realised I would. The fear of it spreading is surely the only fear there is.

It was a horrible moment telling Graham and his wife Kim the news. I waited till almost the last night as I didn't want to ruin the stay. I was also just so bloody nervous. It felt like a confession. Graham is a hairdresser and has seen many clients through it. He was strong and pragmatic. "You'll go through hell. Your hair will fall out. Don't get a wig. Own your baldness.." etc. He took it amazingly well. But Kim told me the next morning that he hardly slept.

We saw Vicky Brown, my surgeon, today and discovered the tumour was Grade 3 – the most aggressive level. She reiterated the course of events – an op, chemo and radiotherapy. It would take about nine months. NINE MONTHS. How could she possibly mean that?

Hi Bella

This is a crazy idea, but go with it and see what you think.

I've just been diagnosed with breast cancer. (Don't worry - I'm fine about it.) I have an op next Wednesday and then 6 weeks later start chemo for 5 months and then radiotherapy. The whole process is 8 to 9 months.

When Johnnie went through cancer the physical changes in him were enormous. At his worst he was a mere 8 1/2 stone. I regret that I did not photograph him. Morbid as it sounds.

So I wondered if it would be interesting to have a weekly photographic record of how I look. For example losing my hair, the scar, my moods etc etc. I may even try and get a breast reduction at the end... If all the photos were put together like a contact sheet it may help others understand the changes that will happen to them through breast cancer. What ever they may be.

Obviously I would have to be naked and I have the hugest breasts. Which may make it an unpleasant photo. And maybe it is something that should only be done with a model rather than an over weight middle aged woman.

What do you think? Is that something you would like to discuss? If you think it is a good idea we would need to get the 'before' photo done on Tuesday.

Let me know if this strikes a chord with you.

Hope all is good with you,

Love Tiggy

Tiggy.

Yes, I would be honoured to do this with you, hugely honoured.

And no it should be done with a normal woman, very real.

Do you want to meet up tomoro and have a chat about it? Or I could do Sunday around midday. It would be good to know your thoughts on the style and how hard hitting you want to be with it. It could be hugely powerful.

Bella
x

18 January 2014

I wish I hadn't told a soul. I am exhausted from replying to emails and calls. I am supposed to be conserving my energy for my op and it has been spent reassuring everyone else I will be ok. Even Johnnie. Following a tiff about whether or not I should visit his spiritual healer he blurted "But you might die." I assured him I would be doing nothing of the sort.

20 January 2014

Despite my confidence of survival I have updated my "If I should die.doc", and Johnnie and I have discussed funerals and wills 'if anything should happen...'

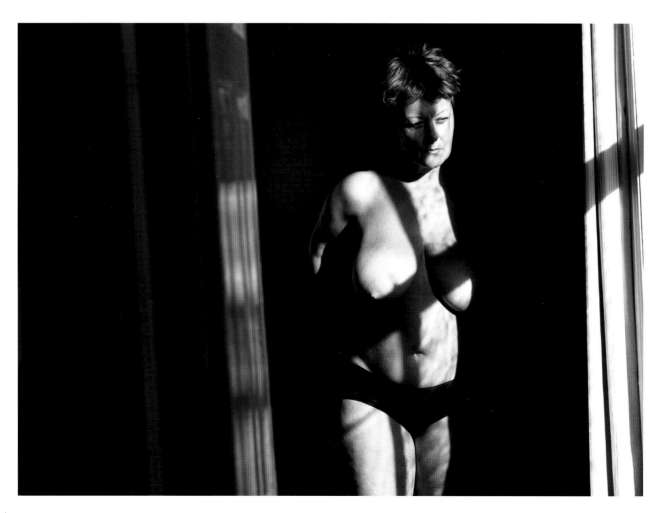

Manor Farm

21 January 2014

"Bella did her first photo session with me at Manor Farm House.
Strange to be taking my clothes off in a derelict freezing house."

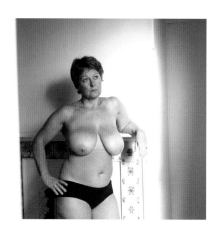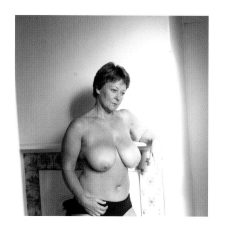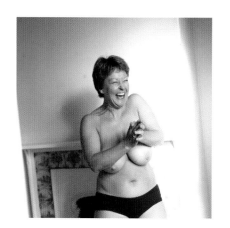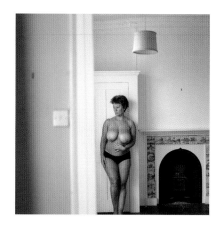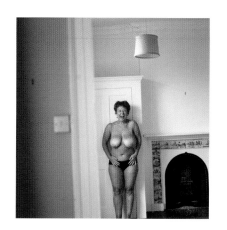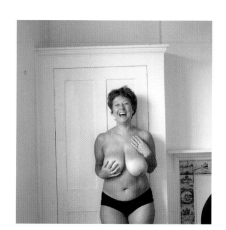

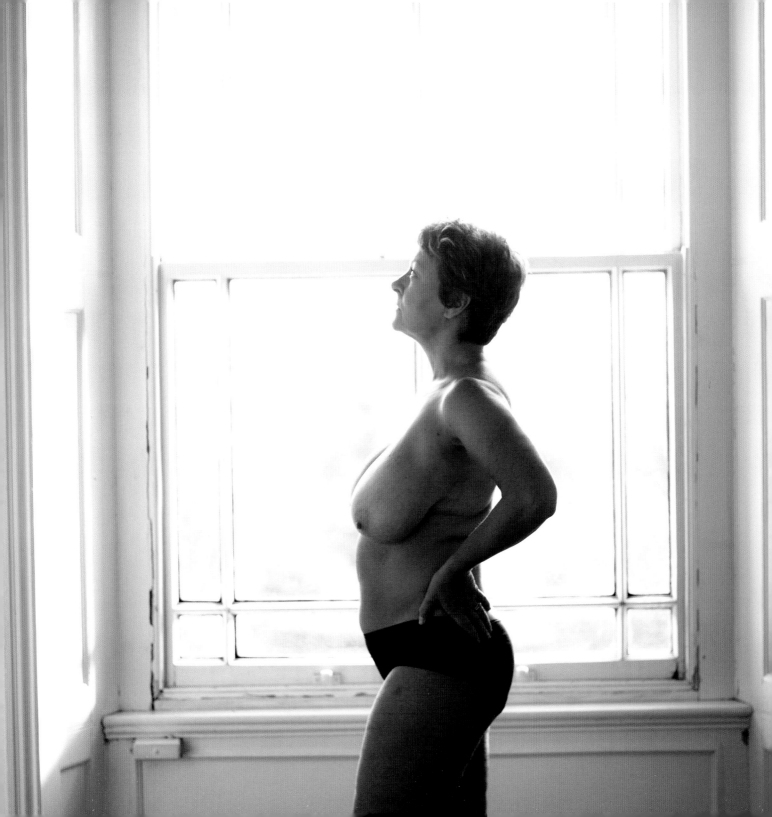

Bella did her first photo session with me at Manor Farm House. Challenging to be taking my clothes off in a derelict freezing house, but Bella loves it as a canvas.

I apologised for the size of my breasts, took a deep breath and removed my bra. She was somewhat awestruck by their size but happily, unlike the Admiral's wine glass, the lens did not shatter and she even made me feel great about them. 'She's good' I thought to myself and before long it felt completely natural to be naked in front of her.

I may not love them, but it is sad to think that from tomorrow they will never be the same again.

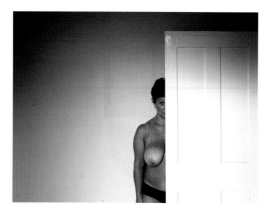
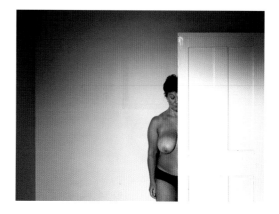
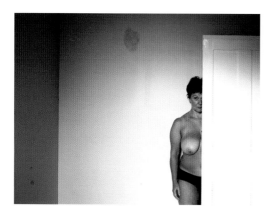
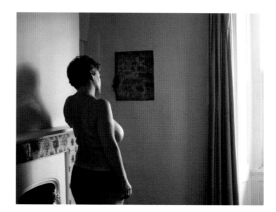

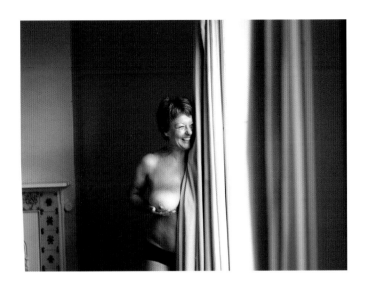
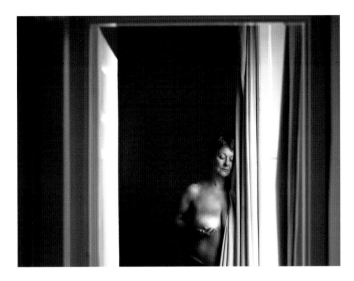
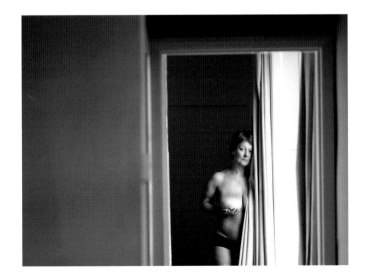
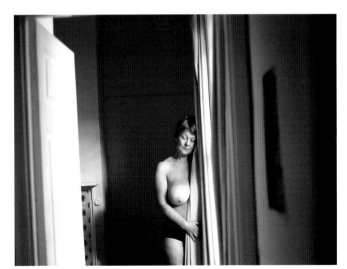

9

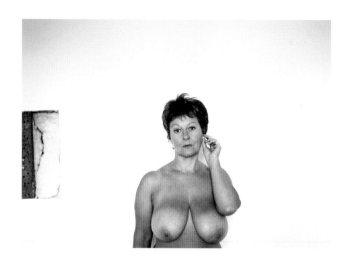
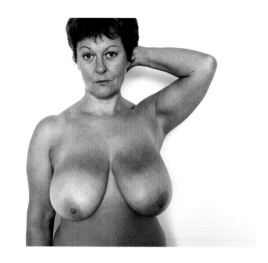
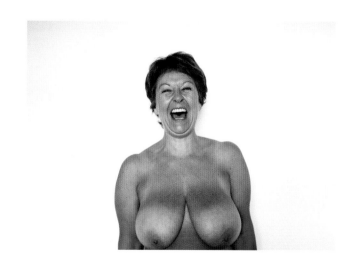
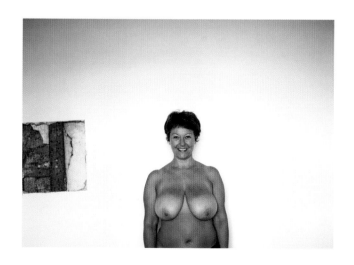

Lumpectomy

22 January 2014

" I never imagined I would walk in to the theatre and hop on the bed,
It was like going for a leg wax."

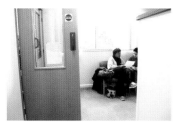
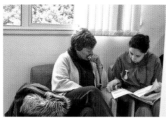
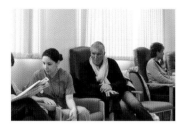
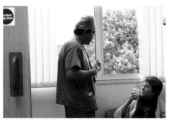
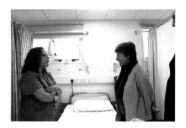
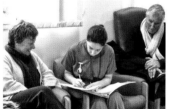
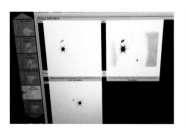
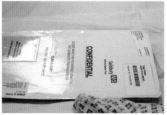
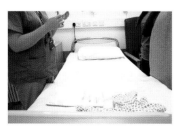
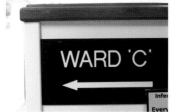

22 January 2014

At last. The day of the op. I was calm. Johnnie was not. He fell flat on his face on the pavement. I offered to drive. He wouldn't let me so I administered tissues to soak up the blood dripping down his hands.

9.30am. The first test to locate my sentinel lymph node which would be removed and analysed during the operation. This would determine whether any other lymph nodes would need to be removed. A dye was injected in to me before being photographed by a huge sort of X-ray machine.

1pm. Admission to the day ward. Surgeon Vicky Brown drew on my breast with a big felt tip pen. Then a wait for three hours while she did her first case. Knowing a lot of people were praying and meditating for me I got in to bed, closed my eyes and soaked it up.

I never imagined I would walk in to the theatre. "Hop on the bed." It was like going for a leg wax. All day I'd been jovial and relaxed, but looking at the vast crew of technicians and surgeons and the huge lights above, a panic attack hit me. Thank goodness the anaesthetic worked quickly. My last words were "Bye bye Bella" as she snapped away.

When coming round my hand instinctively moved to my armpit, "Has it gone to my lymph nodes?". Thankfully it had not.

A nurse asked if there was any pain. There was and within seconds morphine was coursing around my veins. With that and the anaesthetic I was away with the fairies.

Back on the ward Johnnie watched astounded and disappointed as I ate the flabby white buttered toast they brought me. He only got one piece. Before long I was being wheel-chaired outside to his waiting car. "The Archers" was on.

The journey home felt like a drug induced trip. It was. "I love The Archers" I said with all my heart. And then I was sick four times.

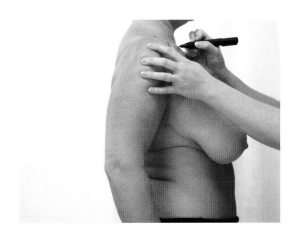

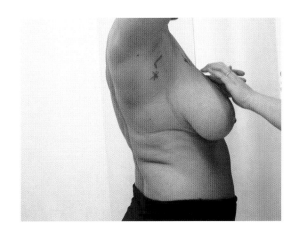

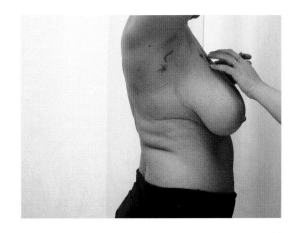

"All day I had been jovial and relaxed, but looking at the crew and the huge lights above me I felt a private panic attack.

Thank goodness I was asleep within minutes. My last words were 'Bye bye Bella.'"

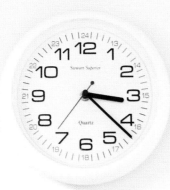

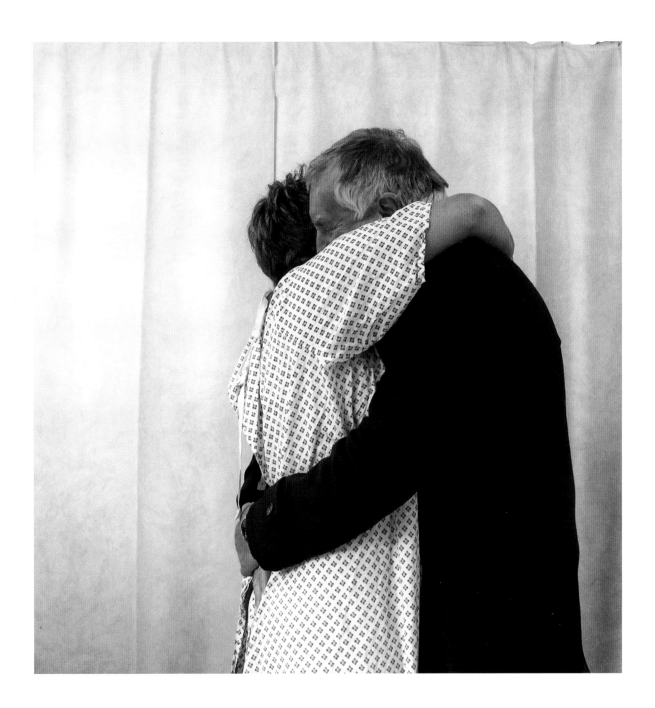

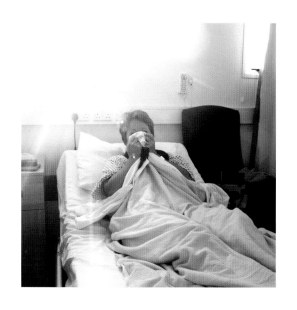

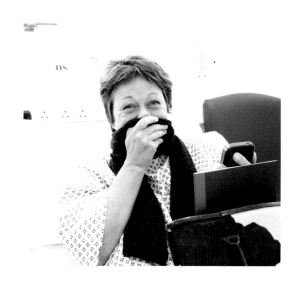

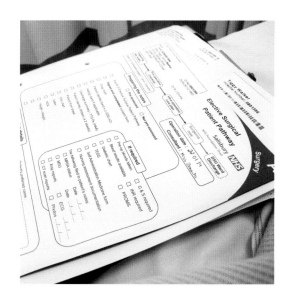

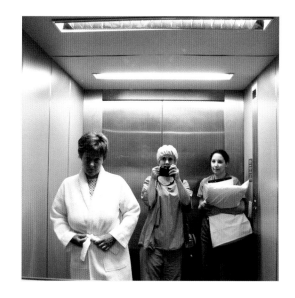

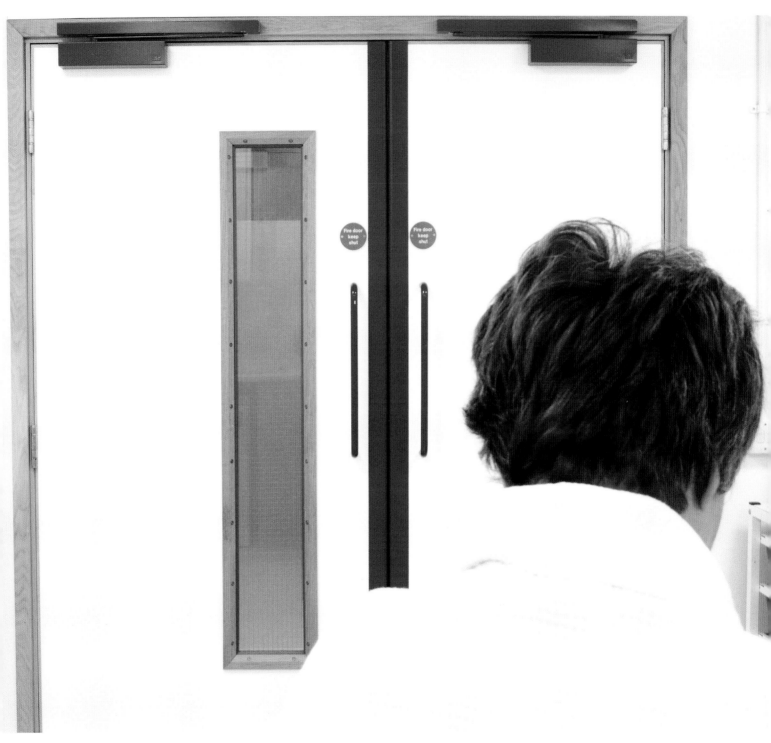

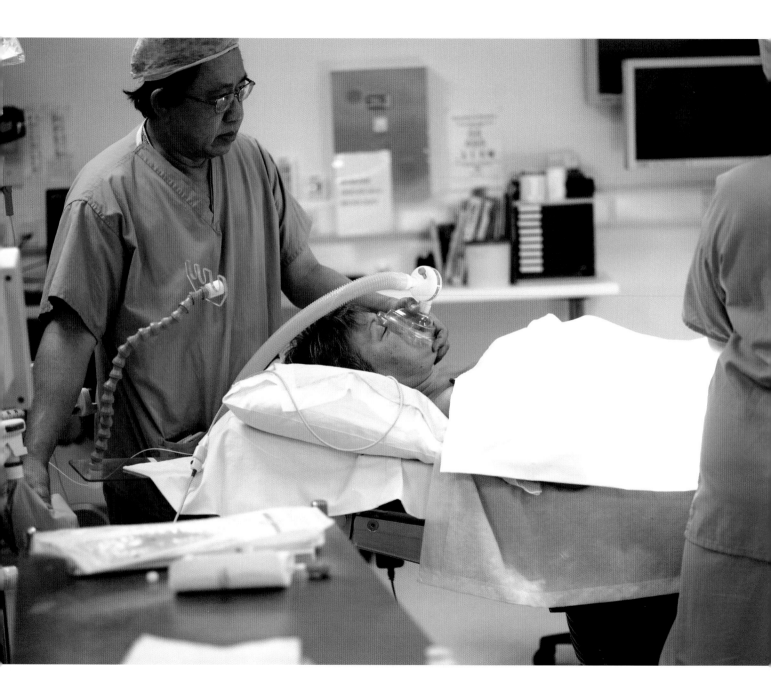

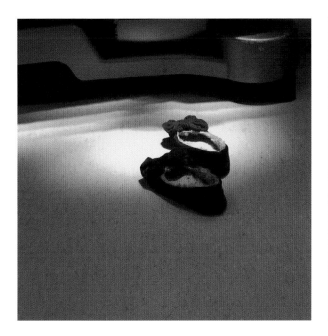
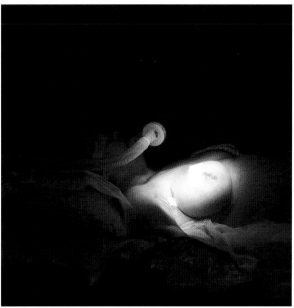

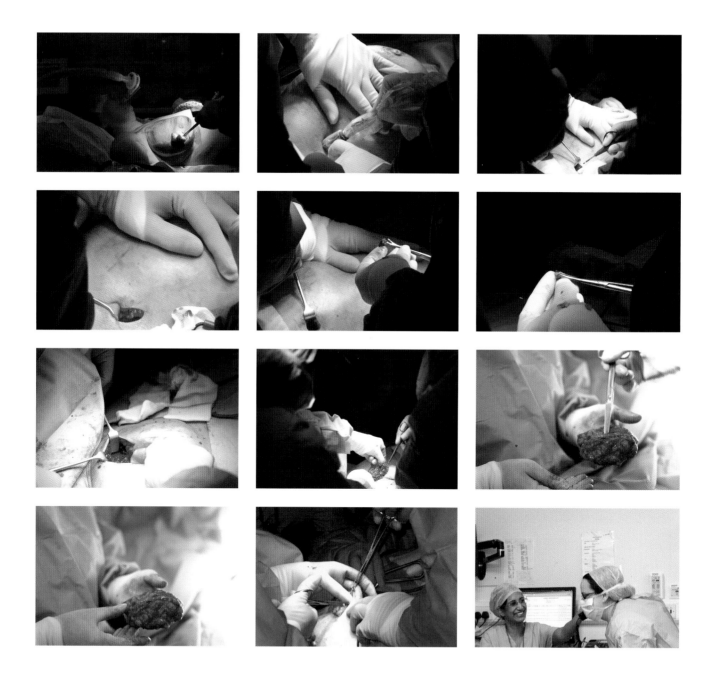

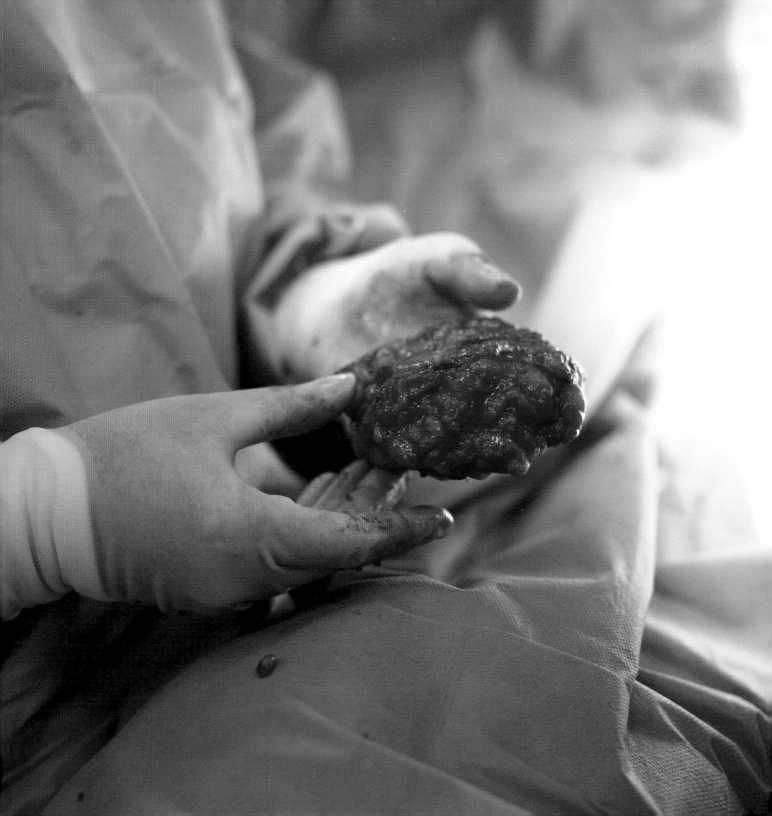

Post Op

23 January 2014

"Mercifully I have no pain."

"My dear friends, family and fabulous colleagues

Excuse the group email but I have been sent so much love and support by you all that I'm not quite up to doing you all individual missives.

I just want you to know that yesterday's op went really well. The size of a small egg has been removed from my right boob. Happily it had plenty to spare so to it only makes a small dent. The great news is that it has not spread to my lymph nodes. This is a fantastic relief. The best news.

Before the op I lay down on the ward and soaked up all the love and meditations you were beaming my way. So calming. Thank you.

My trusted and impeccable chauffeur 'Baines' drove me home last night. (God knows if I'd been private they would have kept me in. It was a monumental effort to get back.) He didn't even flinch as I repeatedly threw up. He simply opened the car door and took the cardboard receptacle, "Let me take that for you Madam."

Once home he became Nurse Betty - walking stick, caterer, hot water bottle filler, drug pusher and flower arranger. He hasn't stopped.

Tomorrow he has to step back in to his more customary persona of JW and fly to LA to interview an 80 something rock chick. (He always has been a sucker for long legged women holding a guitar).

So I will be at my parents for 6 days being spoilt, reverting back to childish ways and learning to knit. Rather a treat.

Thank you again for your cards, emails, texts, flowers, soups, scar ointments and calls. Truly I never realised how loved I am. It's worth getting crook just to find that out.

Next visit on 31st January when I find out the prognosis for the way ahead. I remain an upbeat patient.

My love to you all.

Tiggy xxx"

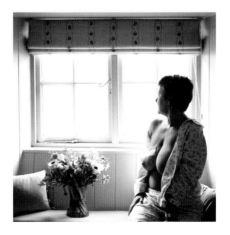
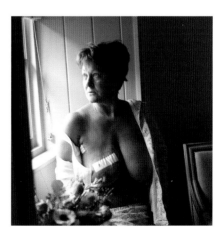

23 January 2014

Apart from the challenge of not lying on my right breast I slept pretty well. I was still stoned. Johnnie and I found ourselves crying with laughter about me throwing up in the car. We were finding the smallest things hilarious. So there is an upside to all the drugs they give you.

Mercifully I have no pain. People never believe you when you tell them that large breasts have very little sensitivity. While this is a huge and ironic disappointment from a sexual stand point, right now it's proving to be a bloody relief. I've not taken one pain killer.

27 January 2014

For the past four days I have been with my parents, Mutti and Pate. Johnnie had to fly to LA to interview an 80 year old legendary female bass player called Carol Kaye. It seemed terrible timing, but in a way it has been brilliant. My mother was born to care. It is her absolute instinct to look after her six offspring of which I am the baby. She and Pate have been amazing. She has brought me breakfast in bed and he has cooked organic healthy meals including the obligatory chicken soup. (I sent ahead strict rules about a cancer healing diet: no sugar, no wheat, no dairy, no red meat, only organic chicken and wild fish.)

When I arrived I felt like a diva. I brought with me flowers I'd been sent, and more awaited me and arrived while there. It was almost festive.

The euphoria dissipated momentarily when by my bed I found a book my mother had bought me: "Facing illness. Finding peace." A well meaning publication about facing your imminent death with Jesus at your side. "I'm not dying Mutti. I've just had an op."

But it did prod my mind. I used to walk with Jesus quite a bit. But with Sunday mornings being about packing Johnnie up to go to London for his show (and The Archers omnibus), I've lost the church habit. It was good to think about the Lord J again.

It is an interesting measure of my concern about my predicament. I have not turned to prayer, yet all those around me who believe, have. It made me realise that I am the person least worried about me.

Post Op Consult

" I got the impression they didn't quite know what caused mine. Stress I told them."

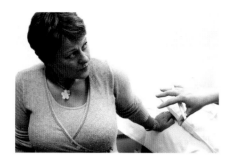 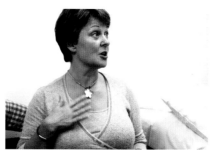 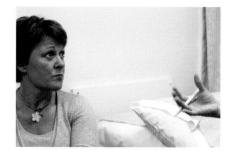

Finally my appointment with Vicky Brown, who very quickly reassured me the op had gone well and that they'd got 'good clearance'. But there were batches of tests that needed re-doing. On the plus side, she said the cancer was not hormone-based which delighted me – but not her. They like hormonal ones as they have the drugs to treat them. I got the impression they didn't quite know what caused mine. Stress I told them.

She told me I would meet the oncologist next week to find out whether I needed chemo. That was a surprise. I thought it was a given that I would have it.

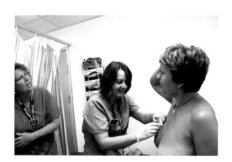 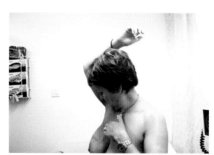 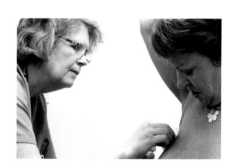

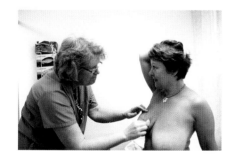 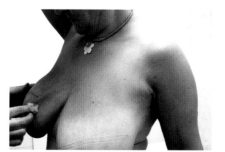 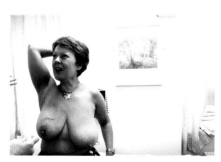

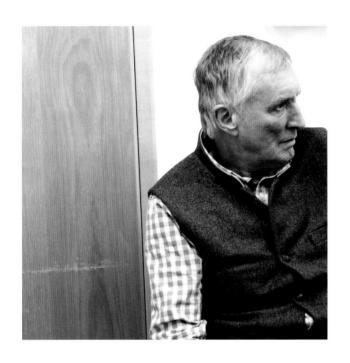
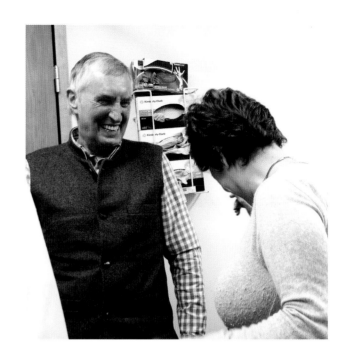
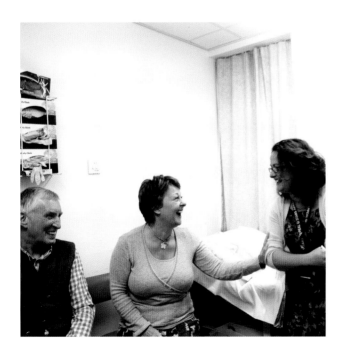
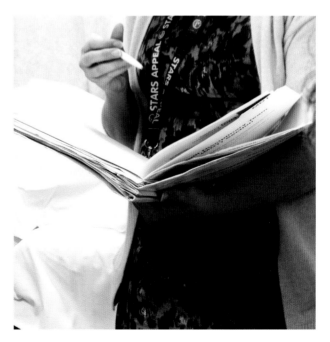

Reflection

8 February 2014

"After so many weeks of positivity – verging on euphoria – I am now in a quiet and lowly place. My energy flat. My emotions closer to the surface."

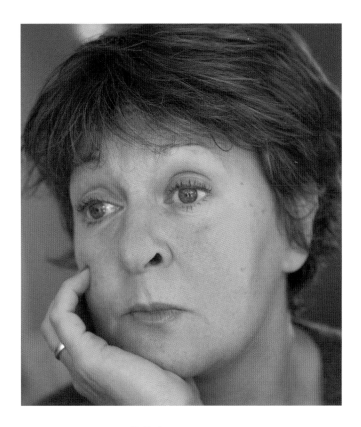

8 February 2014

After so many weeks of positivity – verging on euphoria – I am now in a quiet and lowly place. My energy flat. My emotions closer to the surface.

Last night I cried for the first time since the initial diagnosis. It was only a few tears. Not self pity or fear. But tears of a child who has not had enough sleep. A call from the hospital said my appointment for next Thursday has been delayed by a week. They are still doing tests on the tumour. Of course that throws up questions. I could wonder if they have found something sinister. But I don't. But it will be a month from the op to results which I think is a long time.

What ever it is I am ready to know.

The wait, I feel, is a bit testing.

11 February 2014

Before the operation I had been weighed down by negativity and stress boarding on anger. Now I feel all that has subsided, lifted even. Gone with the tumour. I have this sense of calm and perspective. Everything is as it should be.

Manor Farm Progress

13 February 2014

"We are in the same sorry state, the house and I, but hopefully by the end of the year we shall both rise resplendent."

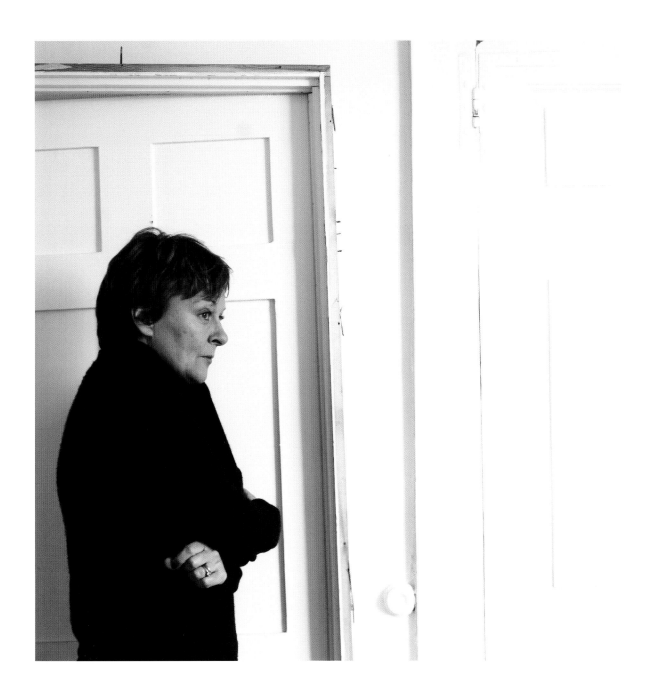

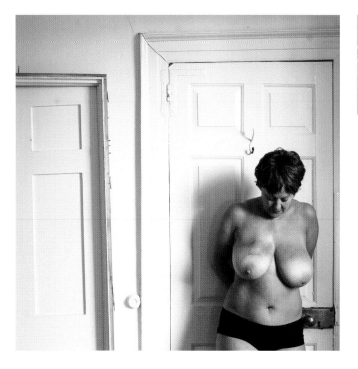
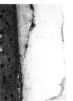
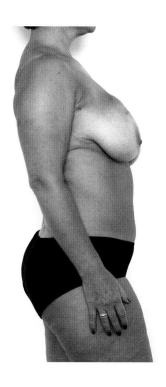

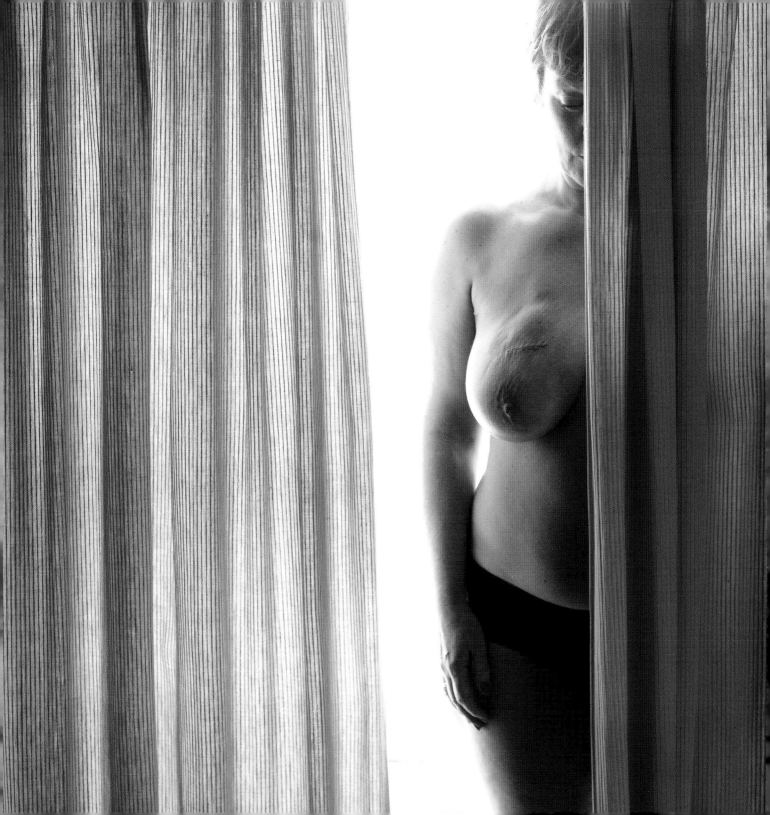

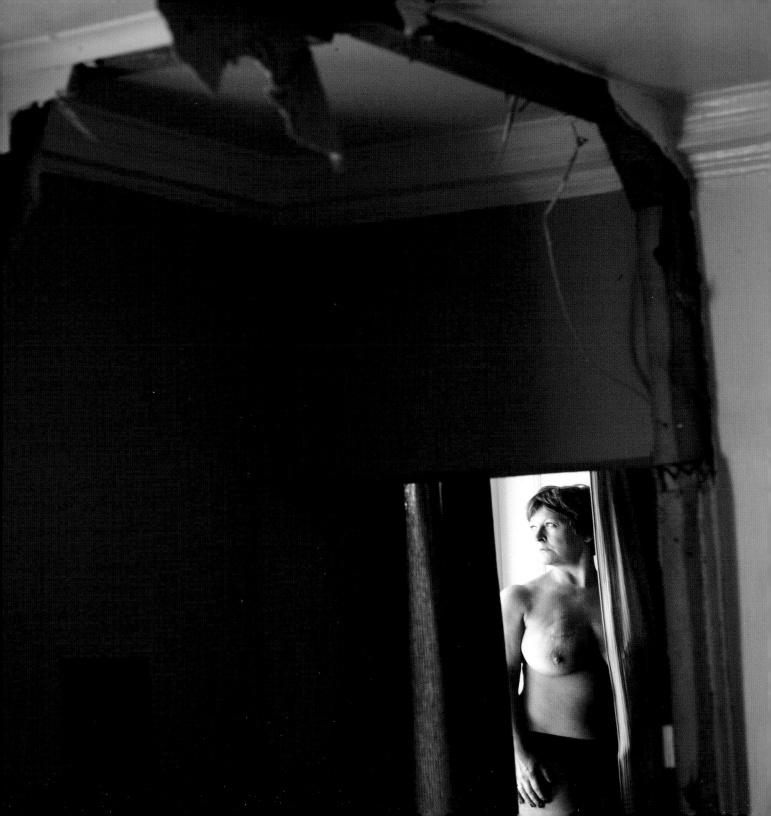

13 February 2014

Another (chilly) session with Bella at Manor Farm House. While it frustrates me how long it has taken to get permission to start building works, it does give us a great backdrop for the photos.

From the first moment I saw this house about five years ago, I fell in love with it. I can't believe it is now ours. We are in the same sorry state, the house and I, but hopefully by the end of the year we shall both rise resplendent.

I love the synchronicity of it.

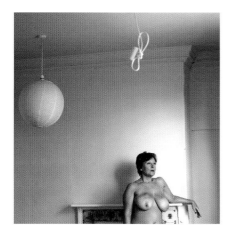 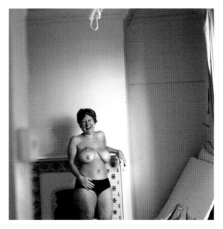 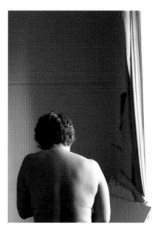 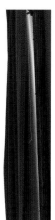

Prognosis

20 February 2014

" I asked all the women in the room what they would do. They would all have it.
No question."

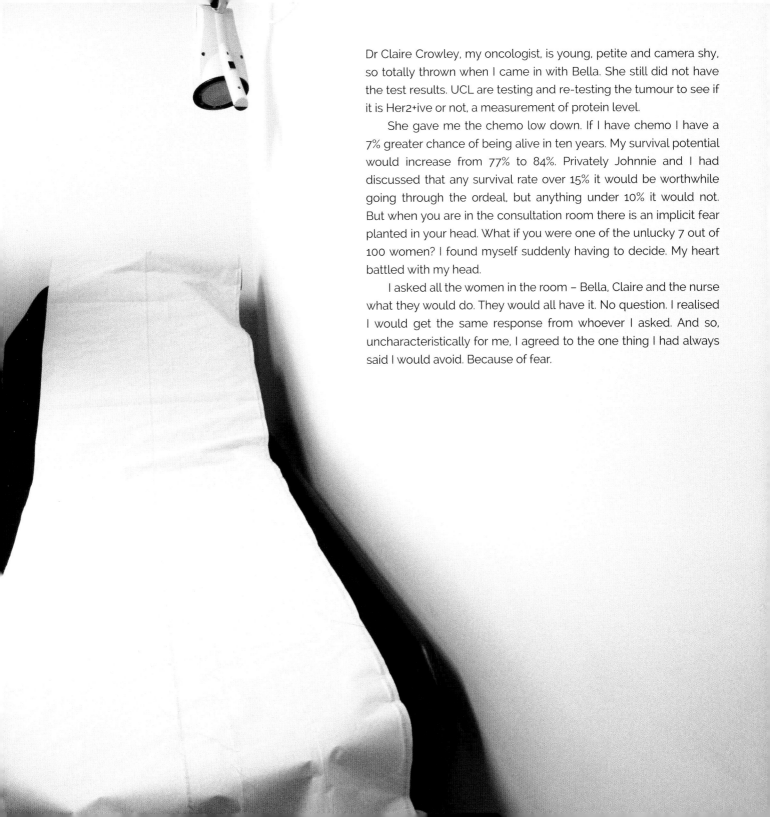

Dr Claire Crowley, my oncologist, is young, petite and camera shy, so totally thrown when I came in with Bella. She still did not have the test results. UCL are testing and re-testing the tumour to see if it is Her2+ive or not, a measurement of protein level.

She gave me the chemo low down. If I have chemo I have a 7% greater chance of being alive in ten years. My survival potential would increase from 77% to 84%. Privately Johnnie and I had discussed that any survival rate over 15% it would be worthwhile going through the ordeal, but anything under 10% it would not. But when you are in the consultation room there is an implicit fear planted in your head. What if you were one of the unlucky 7 out of 100 women? I found myself suddenly having to decide. My heart battled with my head.

I asked all the women in the room – Bella, Claire and the nurse what they would do. They would all have it. No question. I realised I would get the same response from whoever I asked. And so, uncharacteristically for me, I agreed to the one thing I had always said I would avoid. Because of fear.

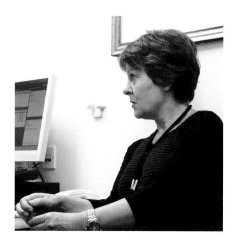 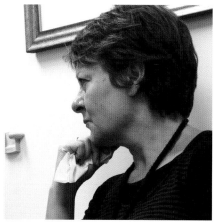 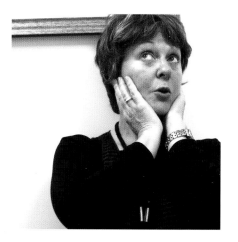

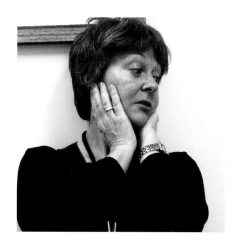 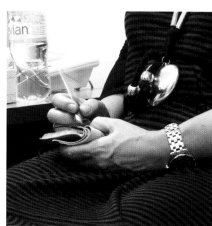 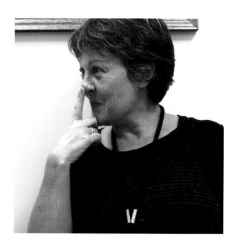

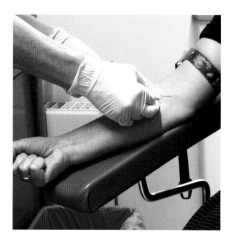 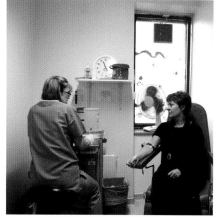 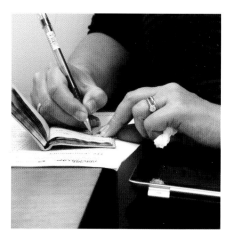

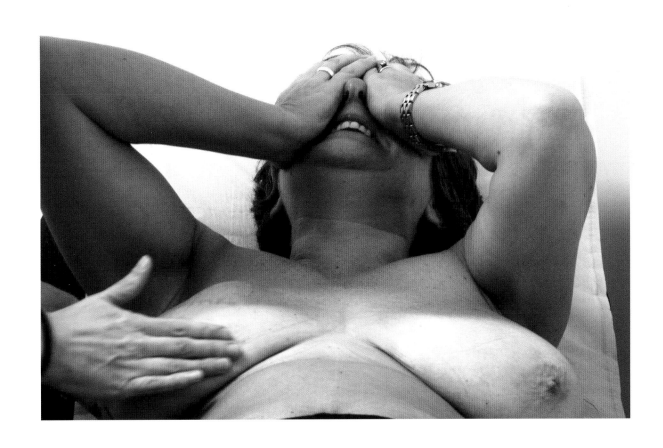

"So my 'lovelies'

Just a quick update for you all. (Yes I am sorry - group email again.) Ghastly. But I didn't sleep last night - worry. So now I know 'what's what' I feel very tearful and pathetic in a relieved kind of a way. Plus I have just discovered that we do have somewhere to move in to in 2 weeks time. Yet more relief. And tears.

Oh yes - the update...

I've been to see the oncologist today and I AM having chemo. Starts 10th March for 5 months. Then radiotherapy after that. I should be done and dusted by some point in August according to my calculations.

They are STILL doing what's called a Her2 test at UCL. But if that comes out positive, it just means an addition to the chemo cocktail.

I am not high risk or dreadfully ill. But the chemo is to ensure it doesn't pop up elsewhere or re-occur in the boob. It was, they reminded me, the fastest growing one you could get. When people talk in terms of your percentage chance of being alive in 10 years, it makes you focus. So I am being good and doing what they advise.

Even though I had started to hope I could dodge the chemo (Cancer? What cancer?) I feel just so relieved to know what lies ahead. I am a Capricorn. We thrive off dates and schedules.

I hope I do not become a ghastly, puking, exhausted, bald and grumpy friend/sibling for the entire time. But if I am, please do not stop loving me.

Love Tiggy x"

Haircut

9 March 2014

"I will be having the poison that I have always sworn I would never have."

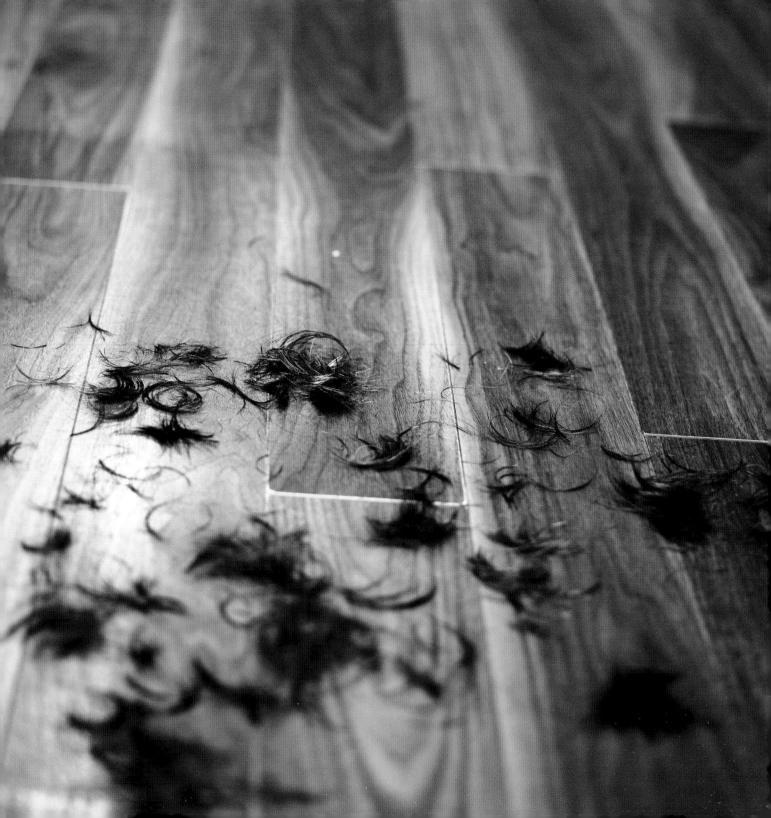

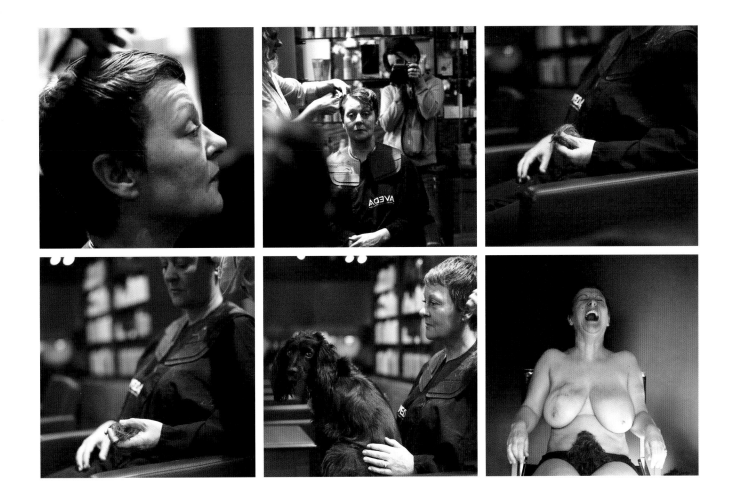

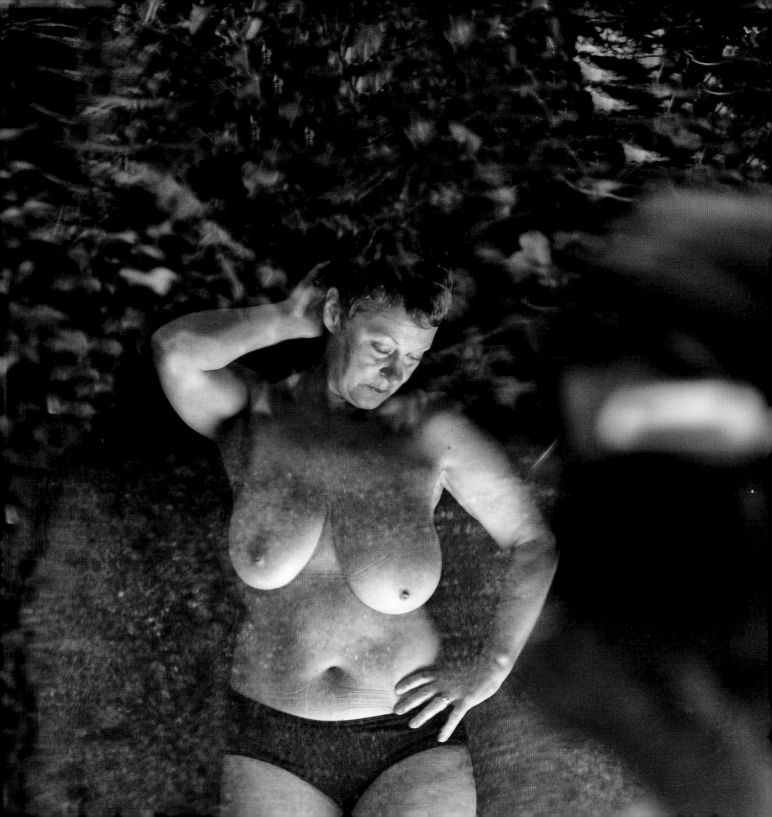

Last week was the almighty and mammoth move out of The Old Fox & Hounds to our temporary home at No 5 while Manor Farm House is renovated. Stuff for there, stuff for storage, stuff for sale. It was a huge logistical challenge.

I've spent the weekend getting No 5 straight. The aim was to build a protective little nest before the first chemo tomorrow.

I went for a haircut with Lisa. There is little doubt that my hair will fall out, so by having it cropped now hopefully the shock will be less wounding.. But it's not only that. It's about preparing myself for a role. Getting in to character. Tomorrow I truly take on the part of a cancer victim. I will be having the poison that I have always sworn I would never have.

It all feels a bit self flagellatory.

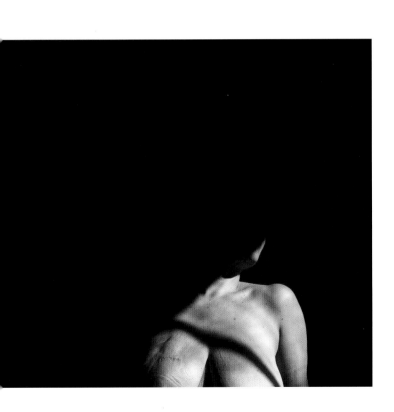
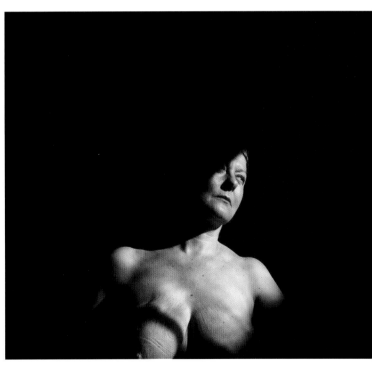

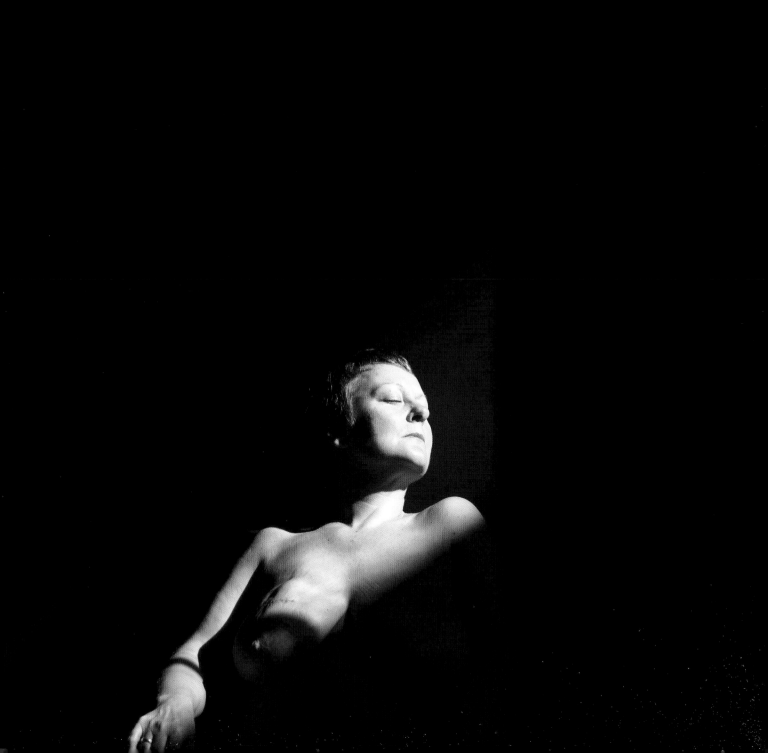

First Chemo

10 March 2014

"As the first syringe of red poison went in to my arm I burst into tears..."

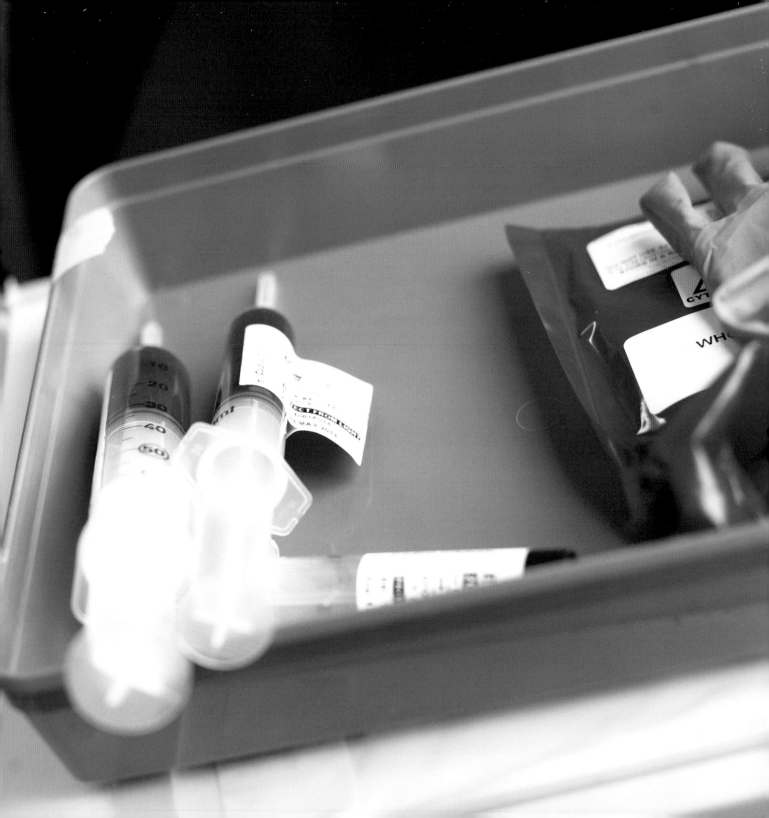

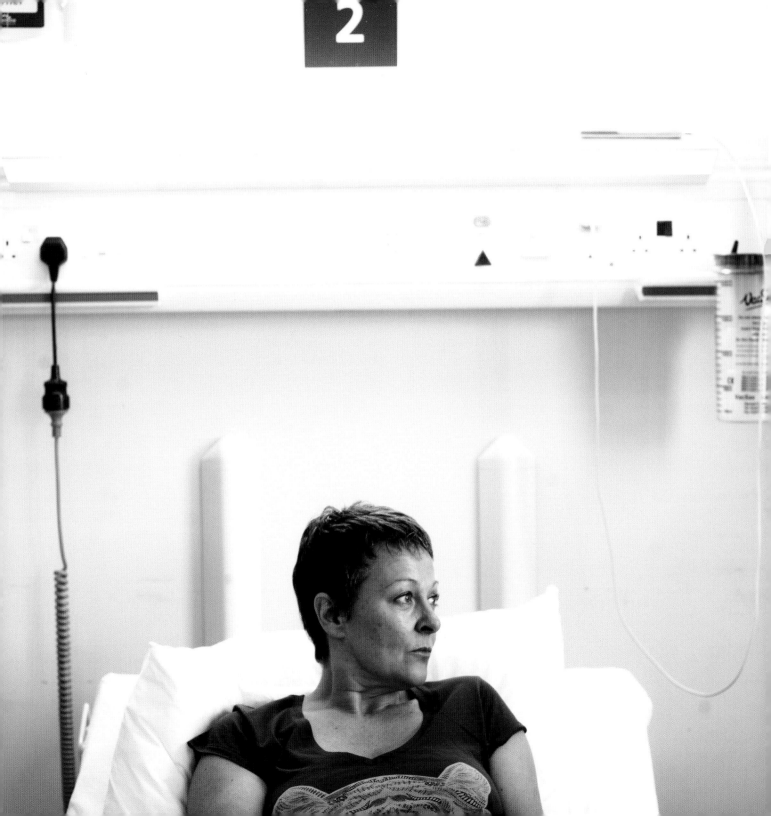

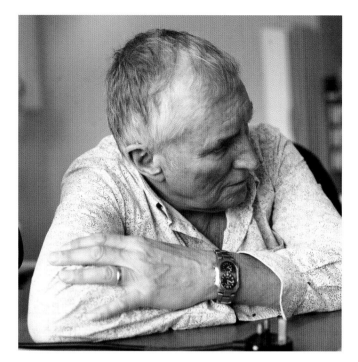
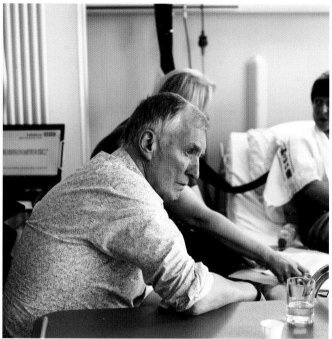
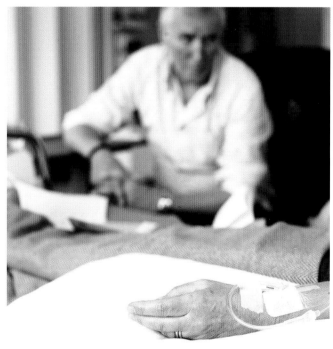
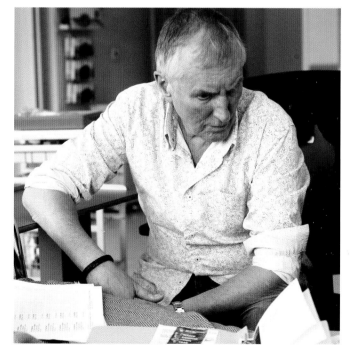

10 March 2014

I arrived tired and discombobulated. Thank goodness I was given a bed. I felt like a lie down.

Nurse Emma, assisted by Jo, applied the cold cap (a freezer compartment for the head to prevent hair loss) while Sister Sue listed reams of side effects, warnings and general negativity about chemo. I was being attacked on both sides by nurses and from above by cold.

Johnnie, Bella and I were having a quite a laugh as I pretended to be engrossed in a leaflet entitled 'Constipation'. But then I saw the first syringe of red poison going in to my arm. I instantly burst in to tears. The thing I dreaded beyond all else – chemical poison – was being infused into my clean healthy body. How fitting that it was red.

We had arrived at 9.30am and left at 2.45pm. Me steadying myself on Johnnie's arm. By the time we got home I felt strange. Within moments I was on our bed crying. It all hit me. The impact of the poison, both physically and mentally, slapped me round the face.

By the evening I felt wretched. I couldn't eat. I felt sick. My head felt like it would explode. I felt like death and out of control. Johnnie held me as I released the most gut wrenching howls. He had never seen or heard me in such utter distress. I was desperate. And I was scared.

17 March 2014

One week on from Chemo 1. What a vile week it has been. The side effects have been varied. Nausea, headaches, unbelievable constipation, hot flushes, feeling cold and incredible fatigue. But perhaps the worst thing is the sense that I am fading away. Not in size (far from it) but in energy. My life force has gone. A dog walk is a challenge, my brain is spent, I have absolutely no battery left. The tiger in my tank is gone. This, with the constant underlying feeling of sickness, has made me sorry for myself and low.

Friends have dropped in to cheer me – and they have. But when they go I am exhausted. Johnnie is limiting visits to one a day. It's all I can manage. I am usually someone who bounces with business and a to-do list. I am a doer, a motivator. But now I am just a husk – and I have become institutionalised. I can't contemplate the thought of going anywhere, even thinking about leaving the house is a terrifying prospect.

I'm sick of these four walls, but I'm afraid to leave them.

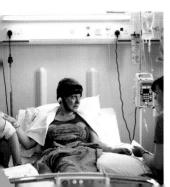 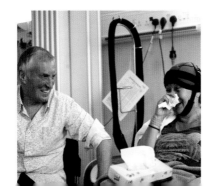 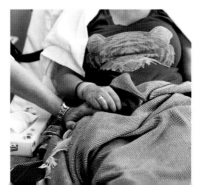 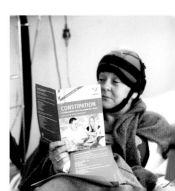

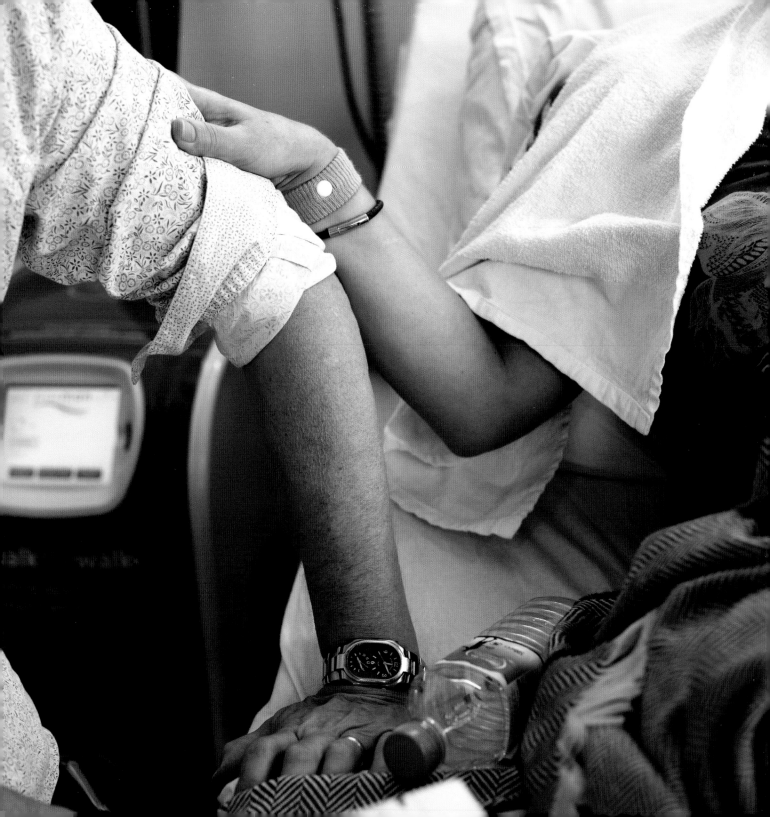

With Johnnie

18 March 2014

"The main battle for me is with my head. I keep hitting myself with questions."

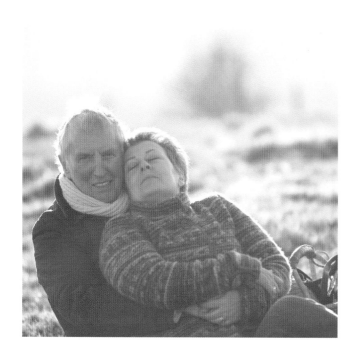
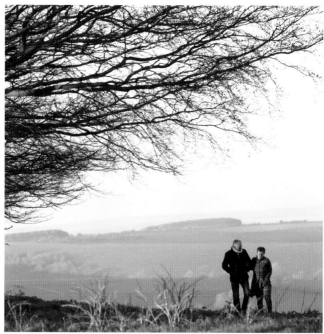

Johnnie listens to every thought I need to share. The main battle for me is with my head. I keep hitting myself with questions.

Can I finish this? Why am I putting myself through this? For 7%? What if I were to stop? Do I even have cancer? It's a real head fuck.

Sonia, the breast care nurse, called and got the full onslaught of my thoughts, unsurprisingly, She offered me psychotherapy sessions. In normal life I would say "No. I'm fine. Don't worry."
Now I was being totally honest. YES. PLEASE HELP ME.

I invited Bella to come with me today to visit Shavata, the Queen of Eyebrows in Knightsbridge, so I could have mine tattooed. I had thought it would make a good picture for this project, but she couldn't make it. I was advised by a friend who knows a thing or two about beauty that it was something I should do before I lose all my hair. It was eye wateringly painful (and expensive) and afterwards I looked like a drag queen.

I hope I shall be pleased when the scabs fall off.

"Hello All

I've had a request for an update. So you're all getting one.

Well, as with life, there's good news and bad.

The good news is that the Oncologist decided that I would only have 4 sessions of the horrid chemotherapy - FEC, and not 6. Not only that but she's taken the F off, as it were, to make it less toxic. So I'm just going through 'ECing hell, not FECing hell. I have this every 3 weeks.

The bad news is that I am Her2 +ive, so I have to have monthly injections of Herceptin for a year after chemo ends. So will all be done by June 2015.

But the worse news is that Chemo sucks. The moment they started injecting it in to me I burst in to tears. I wore a cold cap (a form of freezer compartment on your head to prevent hair loss. Photo attached). I shall not be using that again as it created the worst headache ever. I'd rather be bald than suffer that again. Once home I broke down. I was weak, I felt ill and I was scared. I'd been read a huge list of all the possible side effects as the poison went in. This included the fact that if I fell ill when neutropenic (days 10-14 when the white blood cell count is rock bottom) I would die if I didn't get in to hospital. Charming! That first chemo day was the most horribly overwhelming experience. Poor Johnnie has never heard me cry as I did that evening.

You are sent home with copious anti nausea and anti sickness drugs. The whole combination leaves you feeling ghastly for a week. Side effects abound. But probably the worst thing is that your life force leaves you. As an energy-filled, doing kind of a person, this was very frightening. I thought I was going to fade away and die - without anyone noticing.

The great thing is that after 8 days you suddenly start feeling normal. And today, on day 15, I was back at a 7am circuit training class.

Mentally I have struggled. So much so that when the hospital offered me some counselling I jumped at it. That has been very helpful. I have to start looking at Chemo as my friend. If I didn't have it now and the cancer returned they would be offering me palliative care, not healing. Makes you think.

A friend said that I should get my eyebrows tattooed as nothing looks stranger than a bald person with no facial hair. She sent me to Shavata - Queen of the eyebrows in Knightsbridge. For the cost of a flight to Australia (off peak, economy), I suffered a particularly painful experience, and departed looking like a drag queen. At home a shocked Johnnie said I looked like Charlie Chaplin. Happily they are now fading and people have stopped staring. I'm sure I'll be pleased when the hair does drop out.

Next Chemo is April 1st. Yes I dread it. But the day before I'm having more counselling and having my chakras balanced - as I do. But not at the same time, or by the same person. I will also be more rested as I will not have just completed a mammoth house move.

We are happy camping at No 5 St James Street. And very happily, on the day that chemo started, so did the builders on Manor Farm House. It is fabulous that we will be moving in there after all this shitty period is over. I like it when life works that way.

Sending love, thanking you for yours, and hoping that you never have to have chemo.

Tiggy xx"

Hair Loss

28 March 2014

" My hair is falling out. It spreads over everything – the shower curtain, the pillows.."

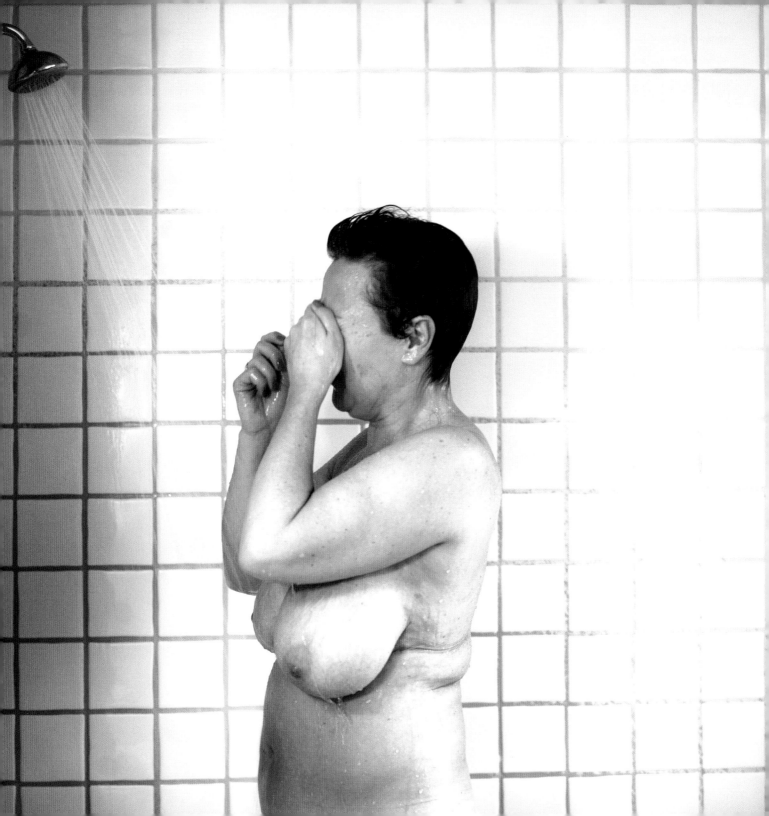

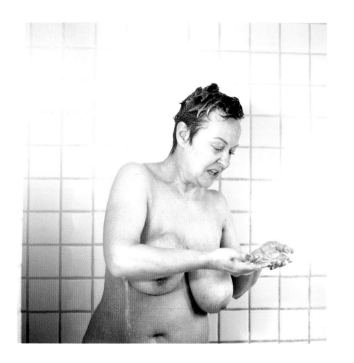
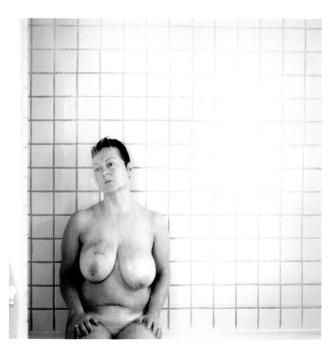
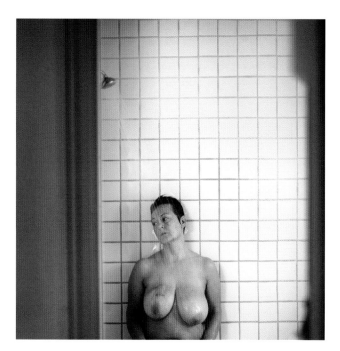
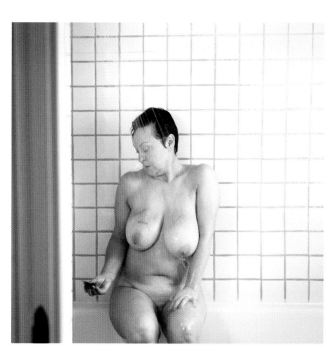

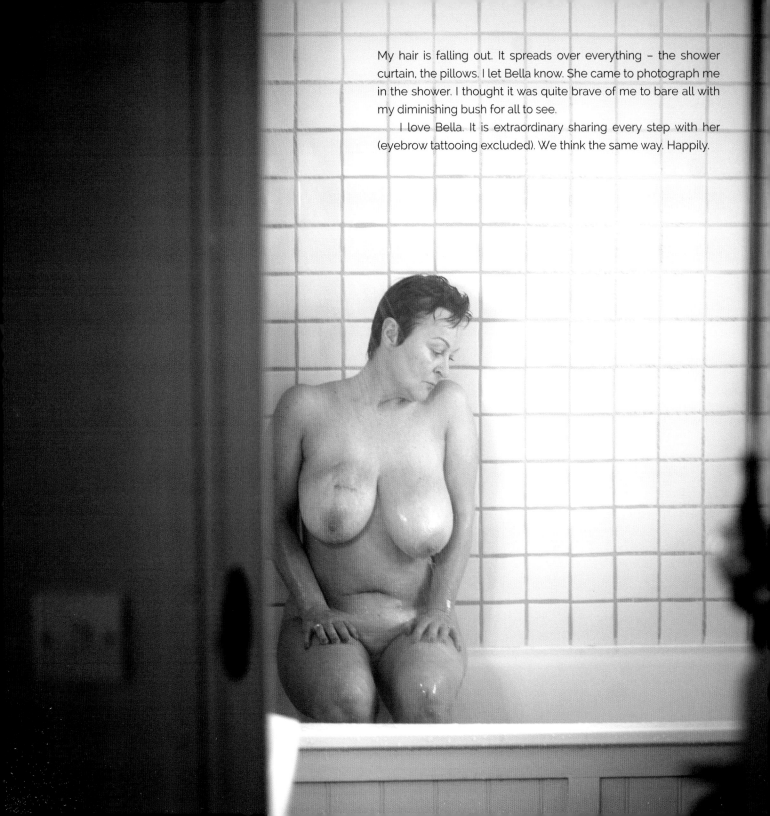

My hair is falling out. It spreads over everything – the shower curtain, the pillows. I let Bella know. She came to photograph me in the shower. I thought it was quite brave of me to bare all with my diminishing bush for all to see.

I love Bella. It is extraordinary sharing every step with her (eyebrow tattooing excluded). We think the same way. Happily.

Healing

6 April 2014

"The needles have released this anger. It had to come out at some point.
If not it would have continued festering - secretly."

6 April 2014

Since an acupuncture session with Salil last Thursday, I feel nausea-free. I have renamed him 'Jesus Christ'.

However, I have gone through three days of tears, emotion, 'why me?' and 'poor me'. I have felt anger. Anger that despite the fact that I am one of the healthiest people I know, I have succumbed to this punitive illness.

I am grateful that by working on my spleen, the acupuncture needles have released this anger. It had to come out at some point. If not, it would have continued festering – secretly eating away at me.

But it has made this weekend unbearable. I sobbed down the phone for an hour to my sister. She is a psychiatric nurse and listened patiently as I told her I cannot cope with the chemo. She'd only called for a quick chat.

15 April 2014

Last week a friend, Abi, asked if I'd tried homeopathy to help with the chemo, I hadn't. So today I met with homeopath, Carole Saunders. What I thought would be a twenty minute appointment was almost two hours.

Bit by bit she peeled off the layers of my onion. I revealed more and more. Everything I could. She had an instant understanding of me that was both reassuring and extraordinary. She will support me through the next two chemos, and after that, work on why I am so sensitive and why my body gave in to cancer. I left feeling so excited. As if she can unleash me from myself.

8 May 2014

The homeopathy is so effective that Carole says it is healing me on a deep and profound level. The reason I got cancer in the first place.

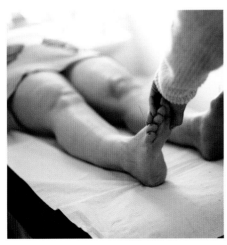 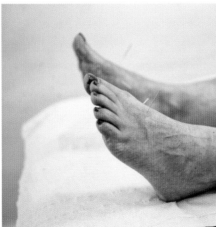 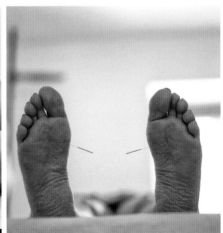

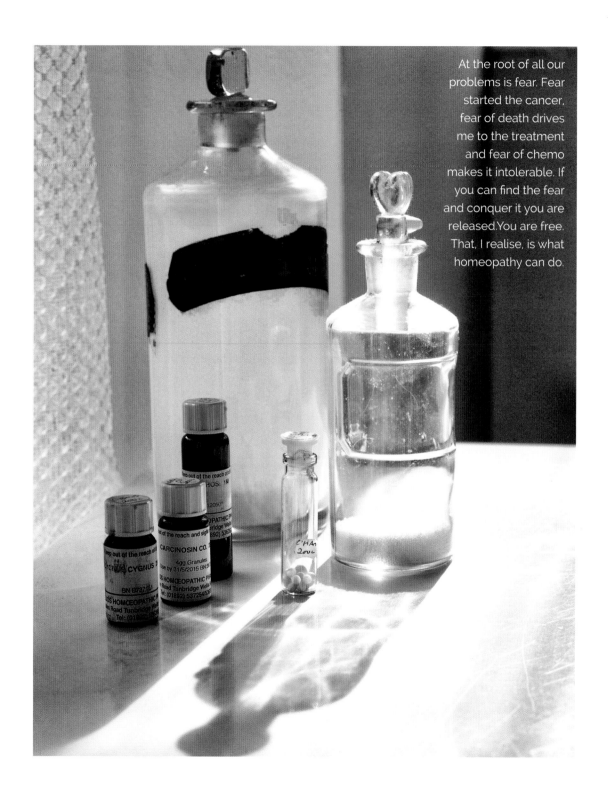

At the root of all our problems is fear. Fear started the cancer, fear of death drives me to the treatment and fear of chemo makes it intolerable. If you can find the fear and conquer it you are released. You are free. That, I realise, is what homeopathy can do.

Head Shave

18 April 2014

" Strangely I was pleased. Proud almost.
This WAS taking control. "

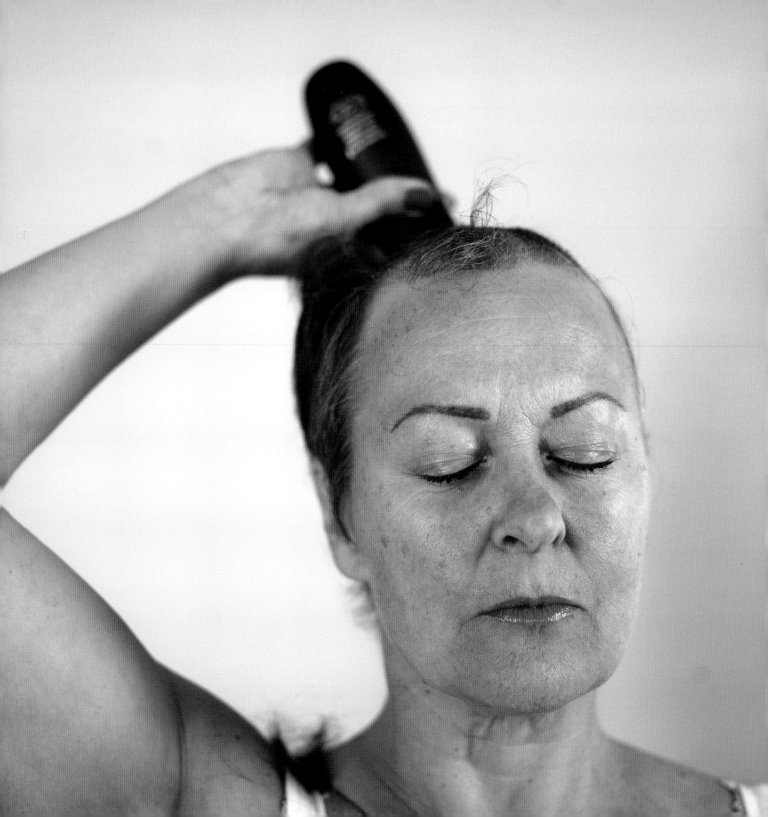

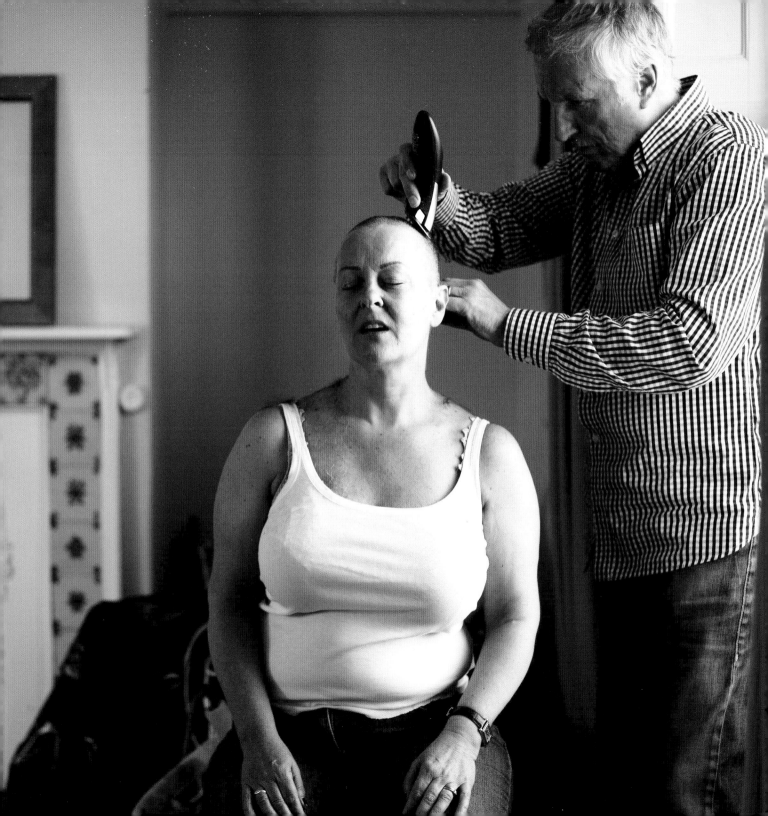

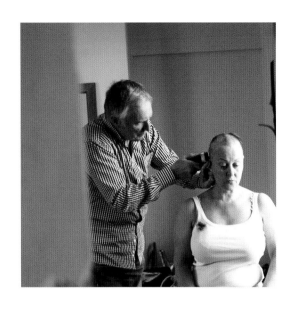
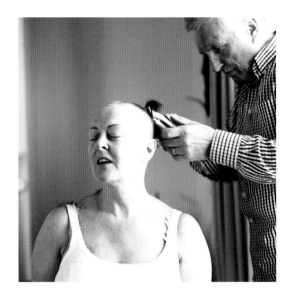
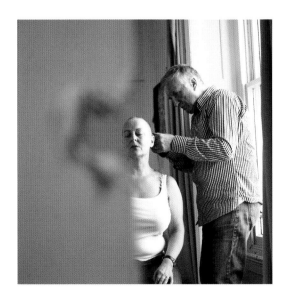
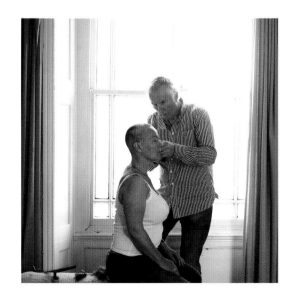

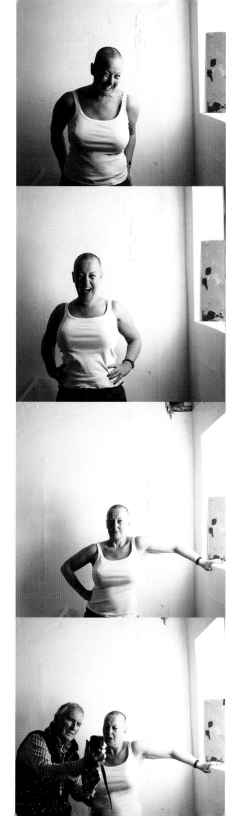

My barnet is noticeably thinner. Bald patches have appeared. Tufts come out when I pull at it.

"Shrinky" (Kate, the psychotherapist) told me that shaving my head was taking control. So today, Good Friday, was allocated as a suitably significant day. If our Good Lord could die on the cross, I could certainly say farewell to vanity.

After a damned good lunch at the Crab House Café, we took the newly purchased clippers to the 'building site'.

"For better for worse..." Poor Johnnie. He didn't know he was signing up for this when we married. He was gentle at first but steadily got bolder. Locks of hair tumbled down. I even had a go myself – just so I could say I had.

Bella and Johnnie stared at me. They complimented the shape of my head. "GI Jane. Sinead O'Connor" they enthused. I felt my scalp. Johnnie picked up a mirror and turned it towards me. "Oh My God" I screamed. I repeated this for several minutes. How I had changed. I've always had such fabulous thick hair. Now just a dark bristle remained.

Strangely I was pleased. Proud almost. This WAS taking control. Now I really looked like the part I'm supposed to be playing – a cancer victim. In that I have been in denial about having cancer a large portion of the time, it is probably healthy for my overall acceptance.

I spent the whole evening stroking my head.

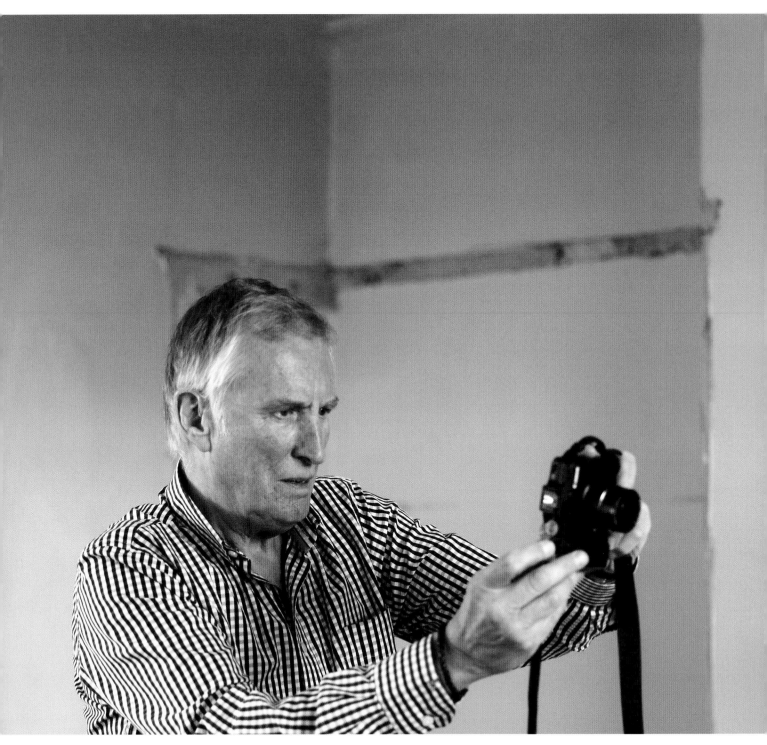

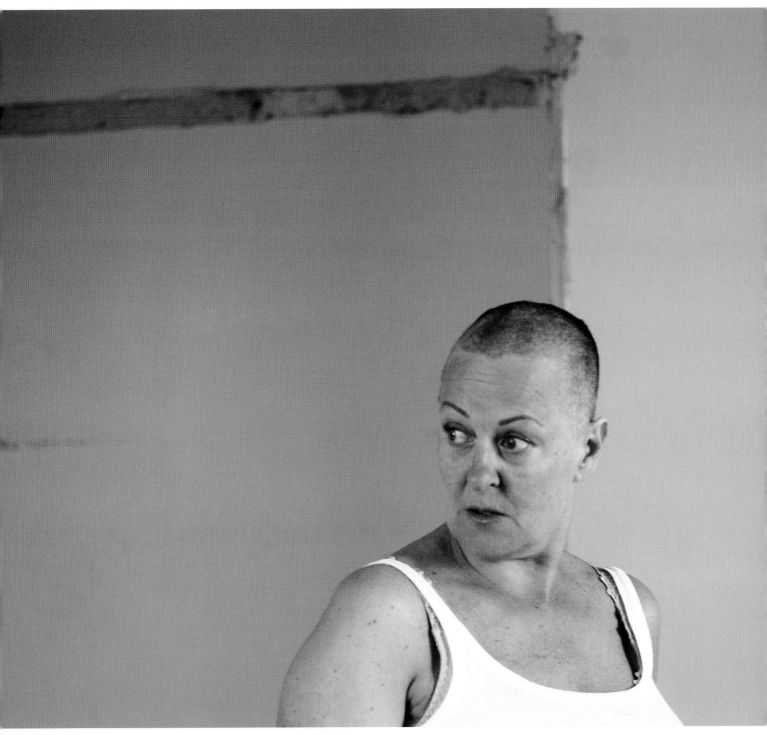

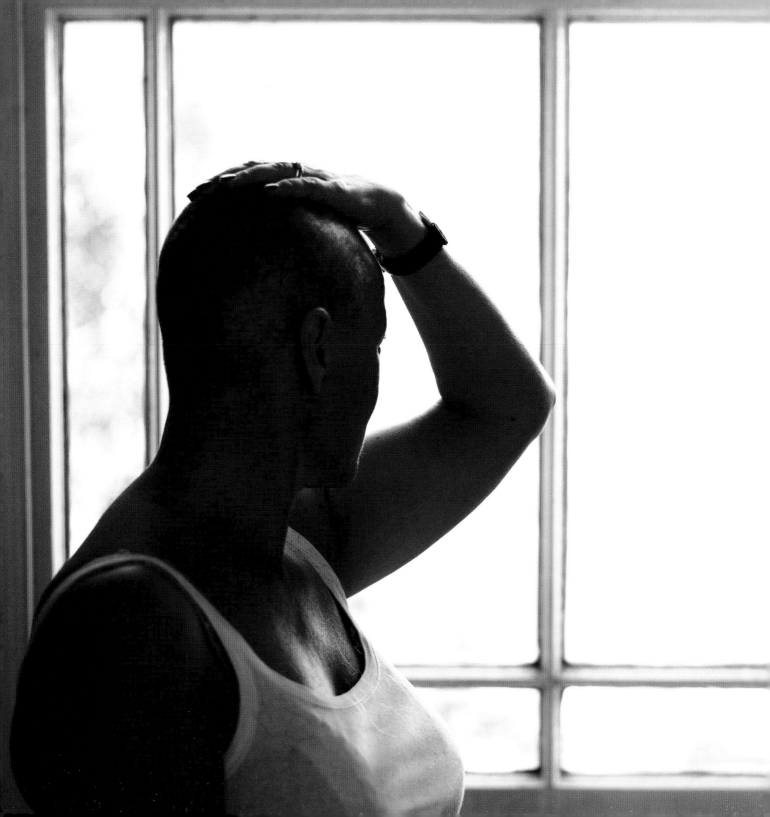

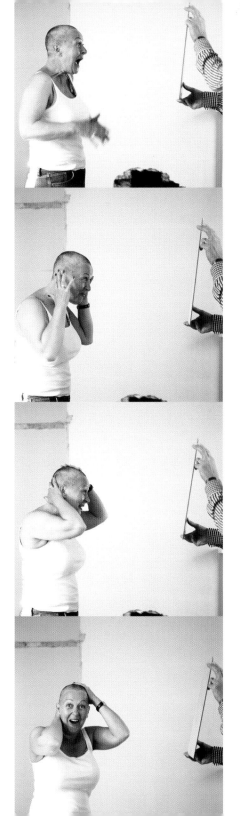

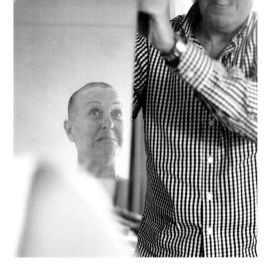

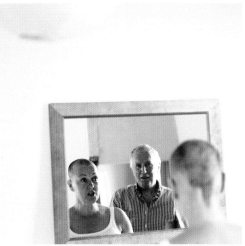

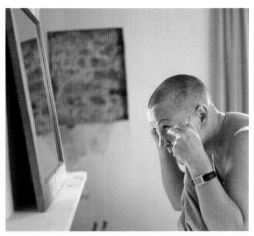

Easter Sunday 2014

Respect to Caroline and Math for doing a stonking Easter roast for fourteen. I had a Liberty scarf that Blink sent me tied around my head. Virginia told me I had never looked more beautiful. The eyebrows were adulated.

By pudding, Virginia and Anya admitted they wanted to see my shaven head. It is the most fantastic party piece taking off your head gear. You certainly get the whole table's attention. And happily I got more admiration for the shape of my head and more Sinead remarks. I don't know if people are just being kind, but they really are making the slap-head look as easy as it can be to accept. Bless my lovely friends.

21 April 2014

It has been a full on Easter. Fabulous that it fell on my 'good days' but also rather over indulgent for one in my state. Especially as tomorrow is the dreaded Chemo 3.

With the fatigue came the fall out. Johnnie and I fought on a walk. He stormed off and I spent the day alone in tears. I realise how hard it is for him carrying me day in day out. Nonetheless I felt justified in leaving a tearful message. "How can you pull a stunt like this today of all days."

He returned but the mood did not ease. I broke down over supper. Of all the nights to be calm I was shouting "I don't want you with me tomorrow. Bella can take me." (A milder version of his own outburst to me twelve years ago when he shouted at me outside Barts Hospital, "It's my fucking cancer. Fuck off." I did.)

I cried and shook on the sofa before Johnnie took me in his arms and calmed me.

Chemo 3

22 April 2014

" I find it hard to write about chemo day. I just want
to blot it from my memory.... "

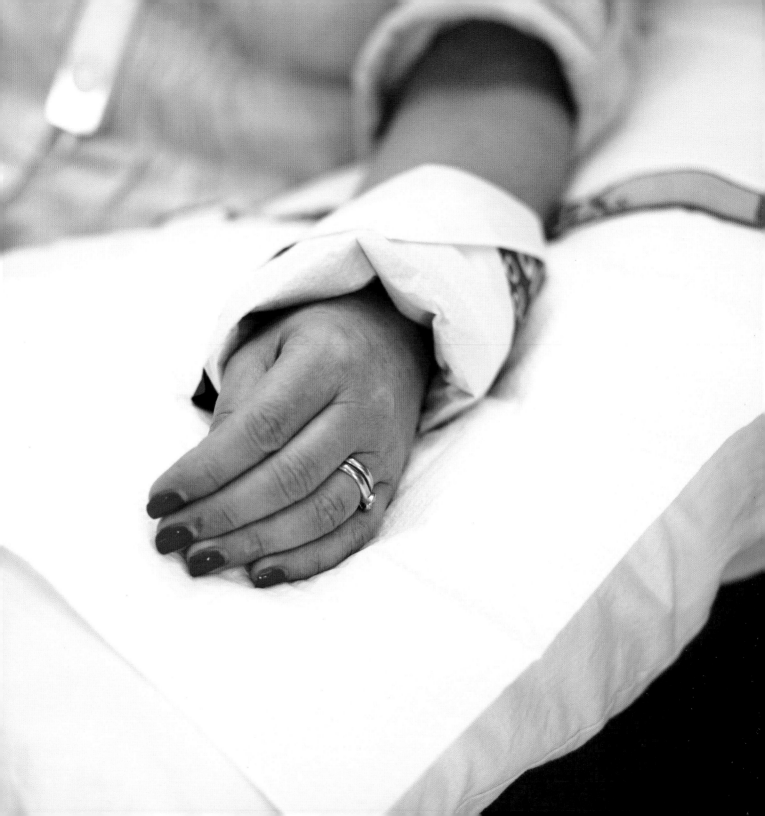

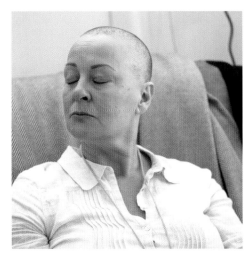 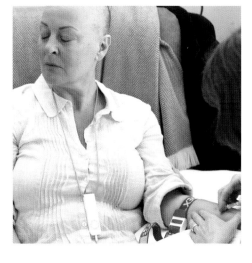

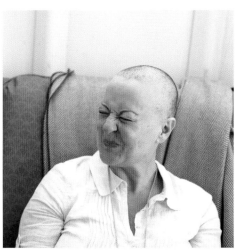 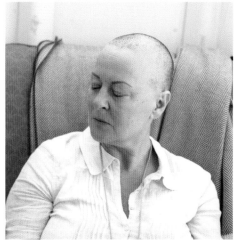

I find it hard to write about chemo day.

I just want to blot it from my memory.

   The first thing you are given is anti sickness pills. These need thirty minutes to kick in, although these in themselves make me feel strange within five. Then you get your 'poison'.

   Today I explained my new tactic. I would not watch it go in. I did not even want to see it. I blindfolded myself, listened to Arvo Pärt, zoned out. Even so I felt tears running down my cheeks when she had finished injecting me. It took an hour.

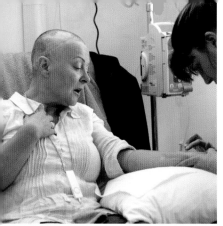 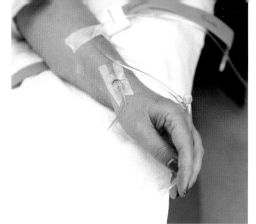 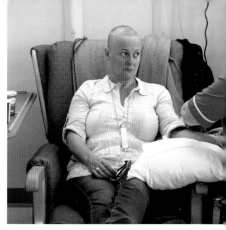

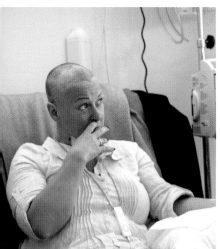 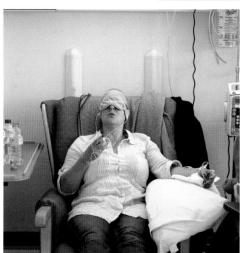 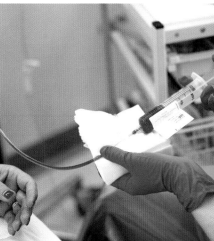

I gave my hat to another patient. An eighty year old lady who admired it but look bemused when I told her she could get one 'on line'. So when I wobbled off on Johnnie's arm, I wobbled bald in public for the first time. But no one batted an eyelid. Not in the hospital.

In the car I tried to face my symptoms rather than mentally block them.

My stomach was burning.

I was very fuzzy headed.

A frontal headache was building.

I felt weak and pathetic.

My left arm was really painful. From the wrist where the canula went in right up to the bicep. So sore. It makes me feel sick that this is caused by that bloody red stuff coursing through my veins.

What irreparable damage is being done?

Squash Court

27 April 2014

" I am so shocked I cannot look at the photos on my laptop. "

27 April 2014

"Are you ready?" The title of Bella's email. No I was not.

I'd asked to see a couple of our shots to send to an agent with the suggestion of a book. This plan goes straight out of the window. I cannot believe the size of my breasts. Even worse – my stomach. And then I see how I have aged. So shocked, I cannot look at the photos on my laptop. They remain small and less threatening on my phone. I cannot reply to Bella or even send them to Johnnie.

I am so disgusted by how lardy I've become.

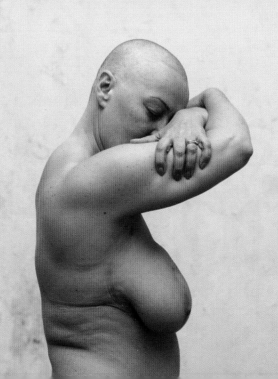

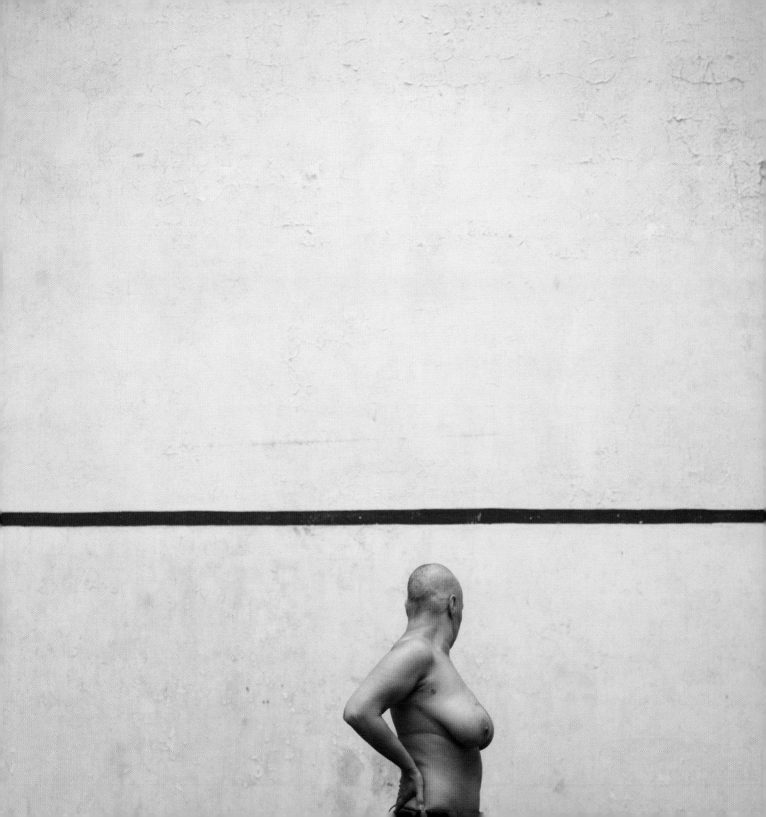

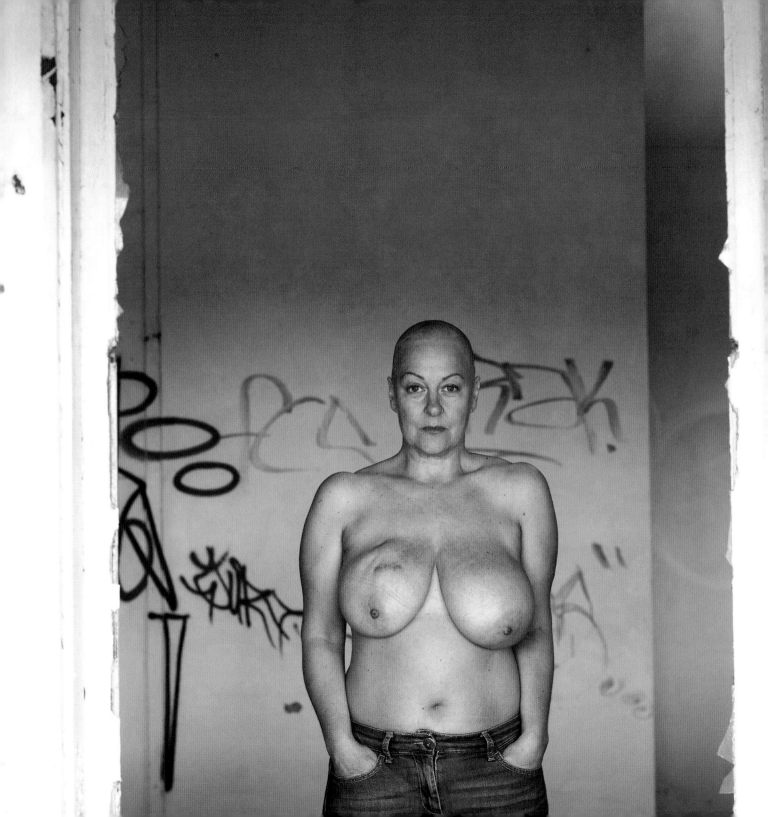

Final Chemo

13 May 2014

" Well it may be the last one but it doesn't mean I
am not nervous and on edge."

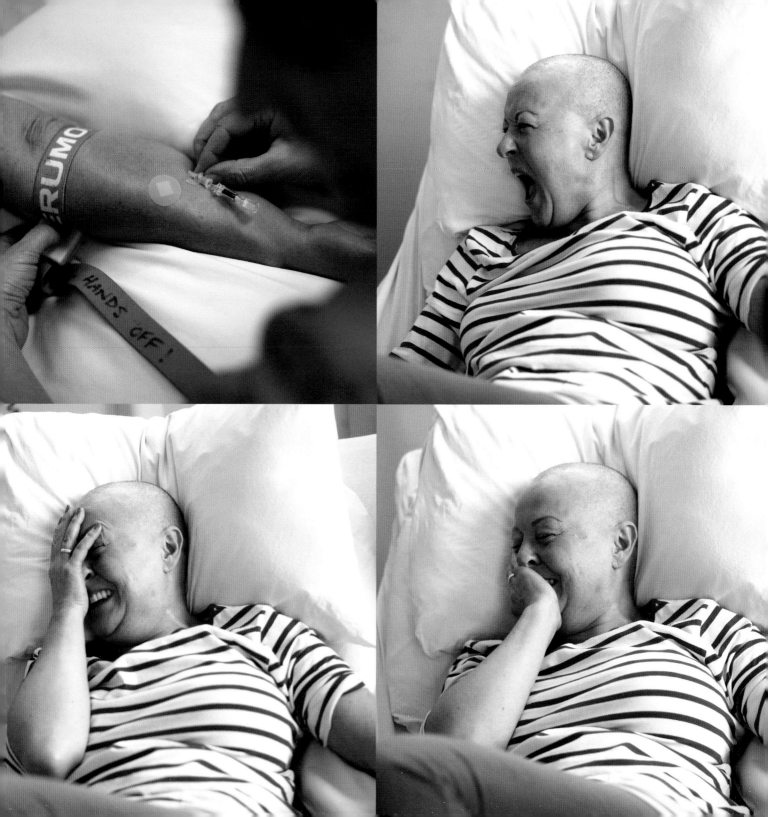

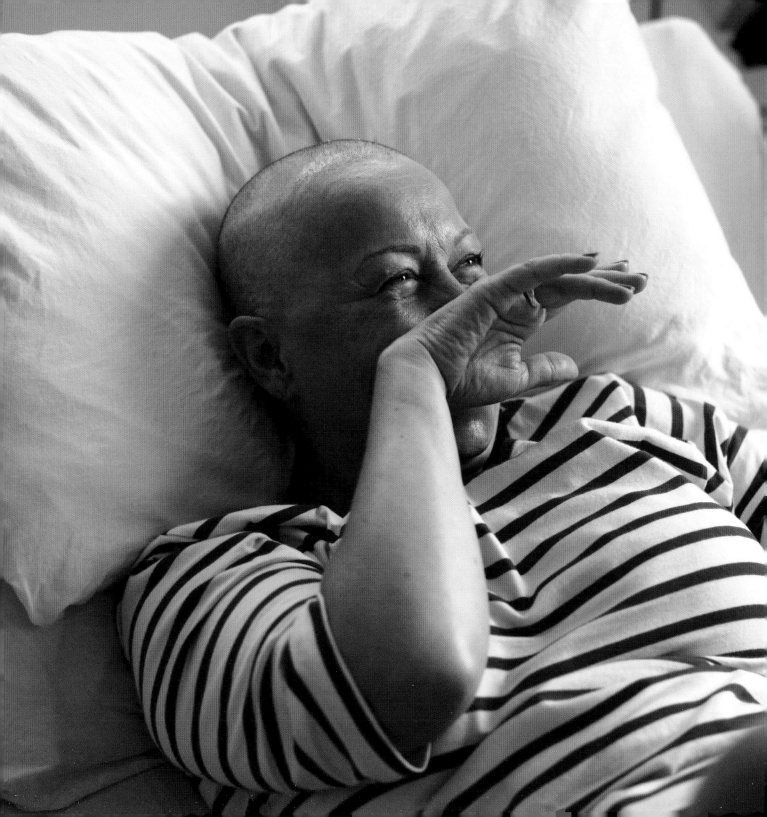

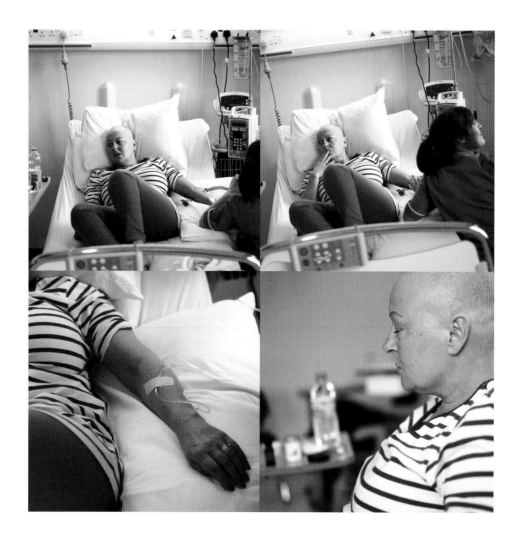

Well it may be the last one but it doesn't mean I am not nervous and on edge. I am almost tearful.. God – I hope I don't freak out and miss it. That happened to a friend of ours last week. She ended up having sedatives instead of chemo.

Johnnie is wisely giving me a wide berth this morning.

I know I'm on edge when I shout "Fucking leave me alone" each time a good luck text pings on to the phone. It's just not balanced.

It may be my perverse sense of humour but I have elected to wear a red striped top. Very themed.

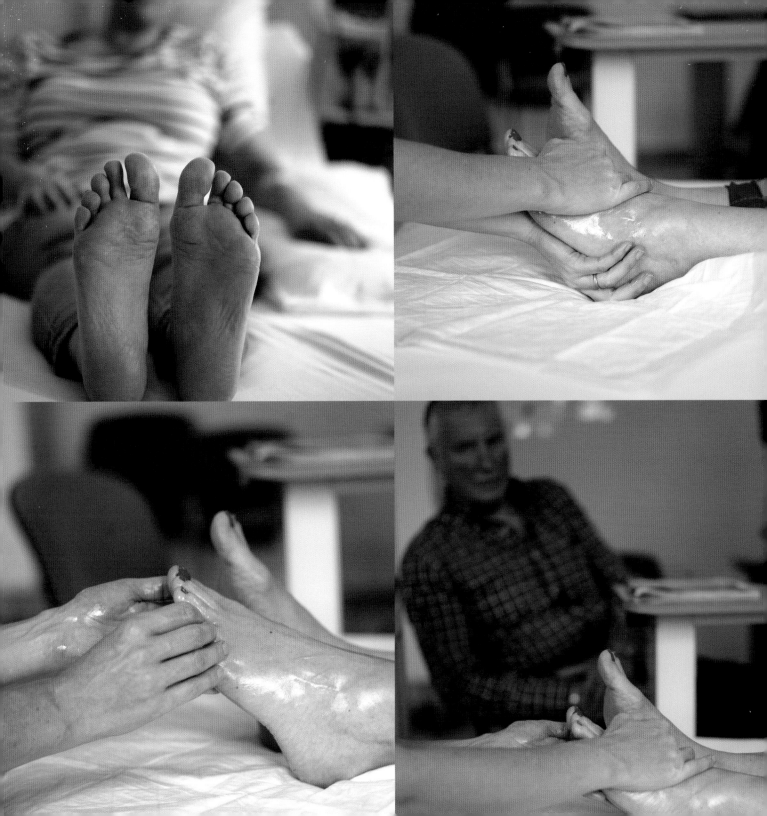

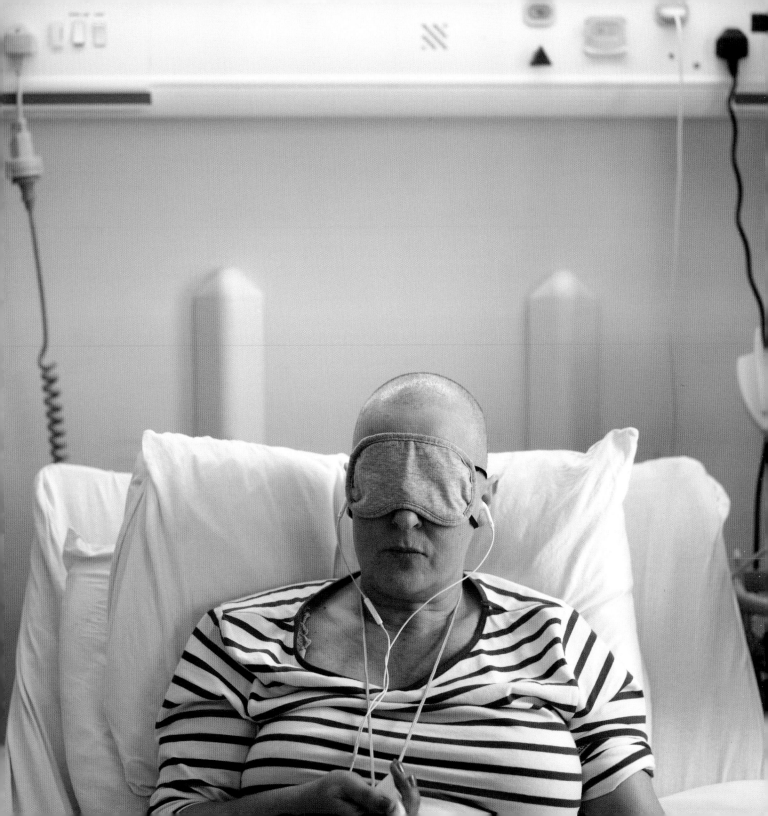

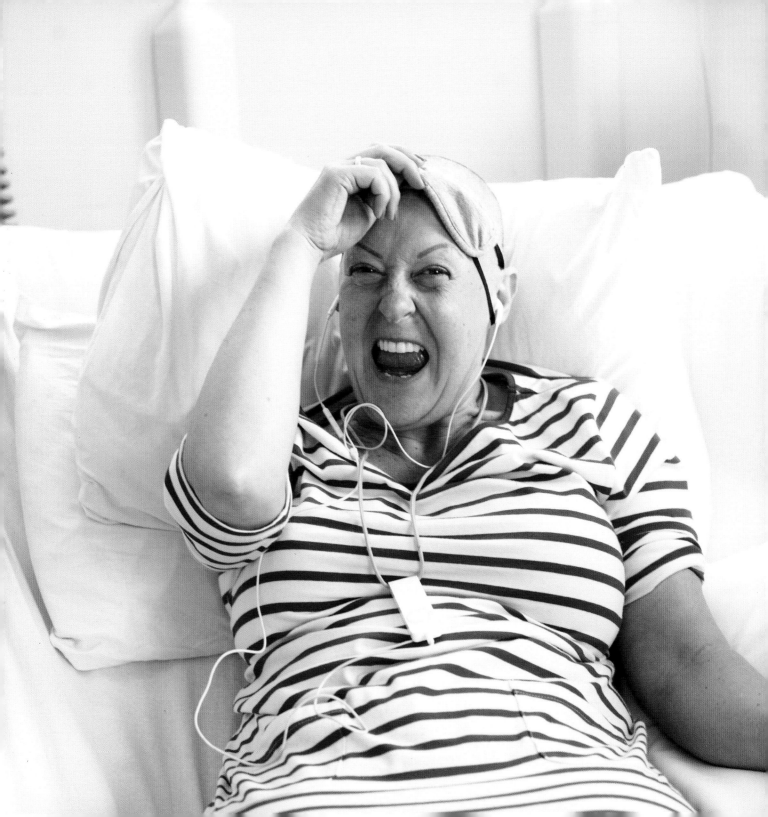

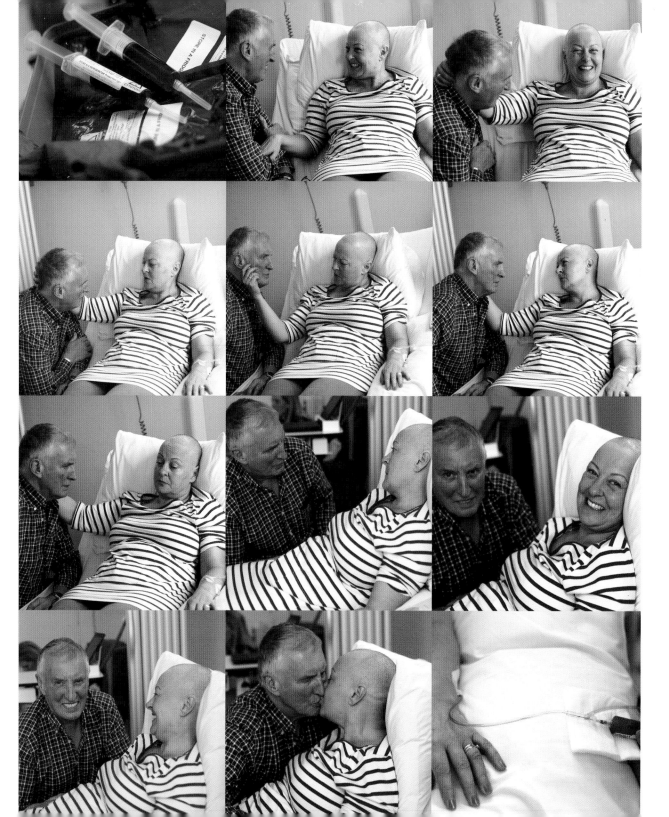

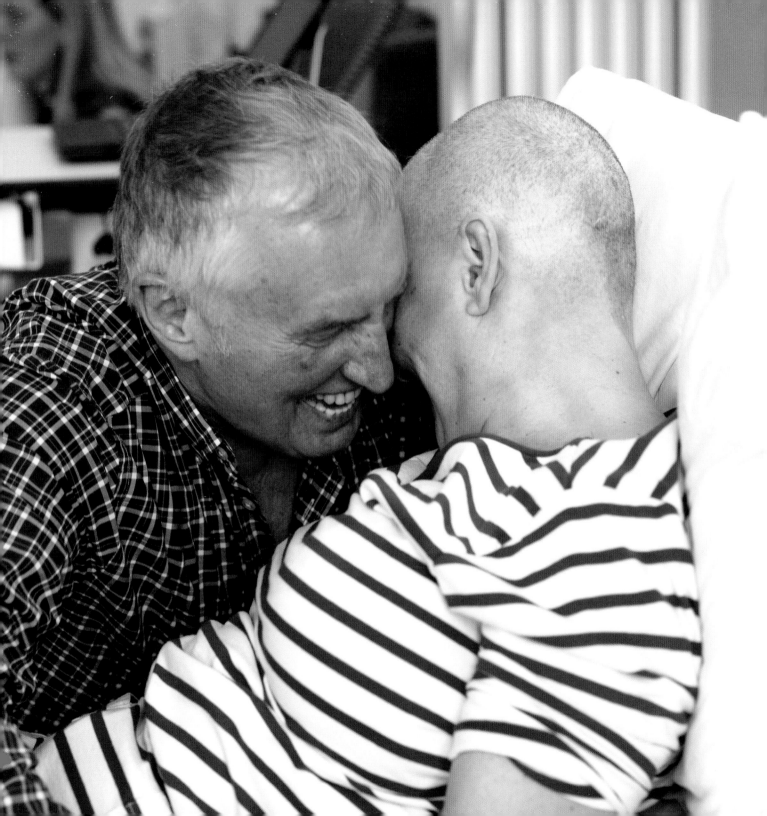

Post Chemo

19 May 2014

" My body was so weak.
I have never had as little energy."

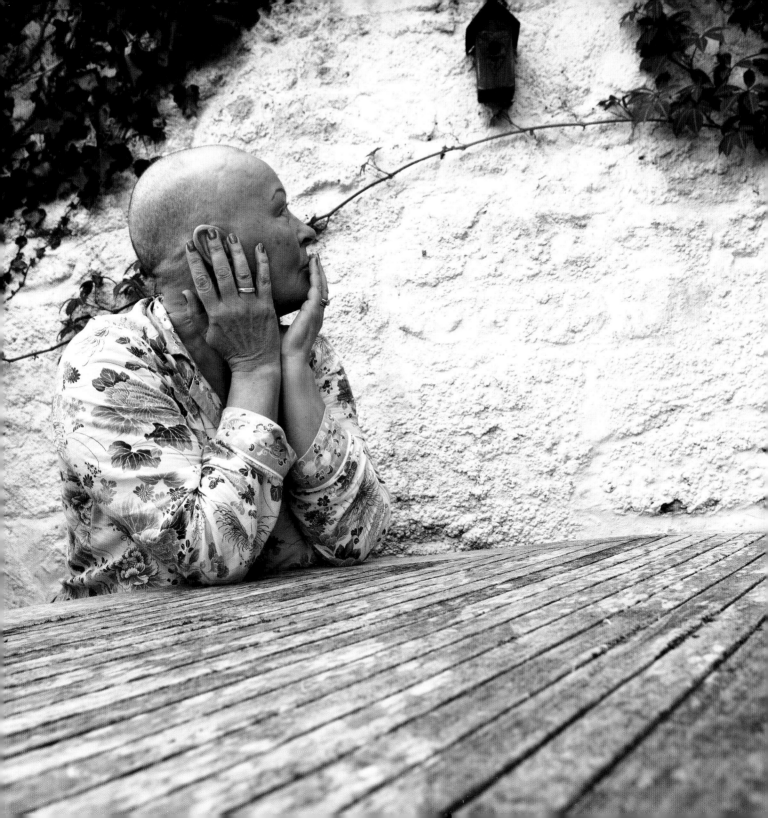

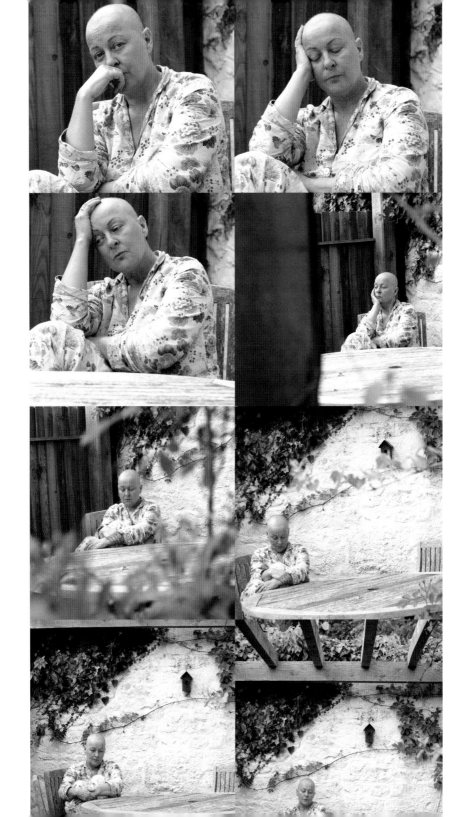

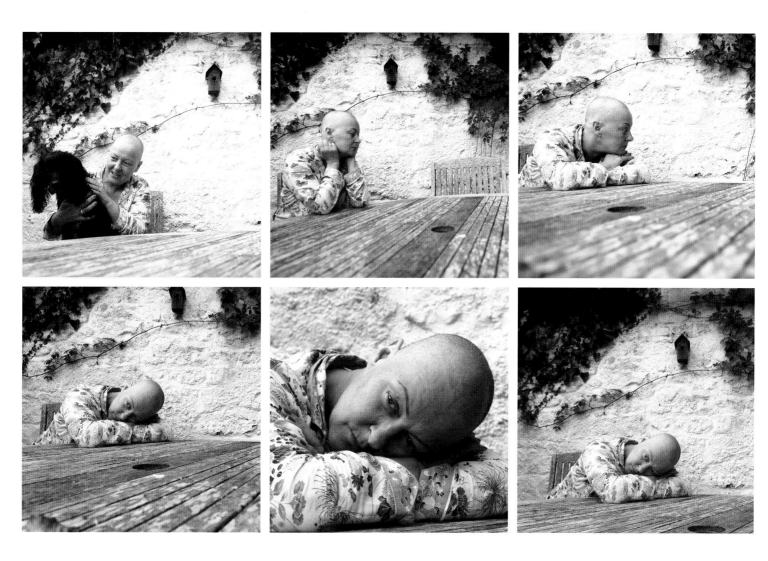

19 May 2014

It has taken me a week and a day to write again. I did very nearly walk out of the final chemo. It took them over twenty five minutes to get in to a vein. Even Johnnie was on the verge of saying 'let's forget it'. Instead he said "Think of Jamaica and a rum punch!" and in it went.

    I slept for the following three days. None of the other sessions have hit me as hard physically as this one. My body was so weak. I have never had as little energy. On Thursday night I asked Johnnie if he thought I would wake in the morning.

    I was running out of life force.

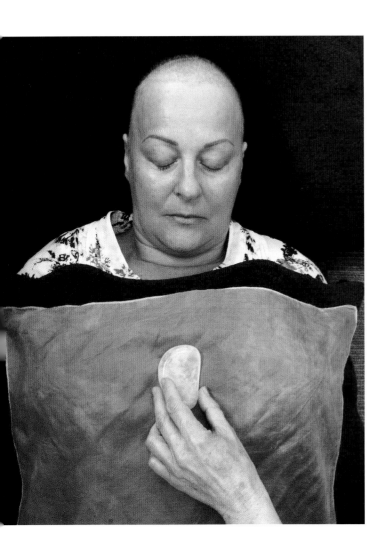
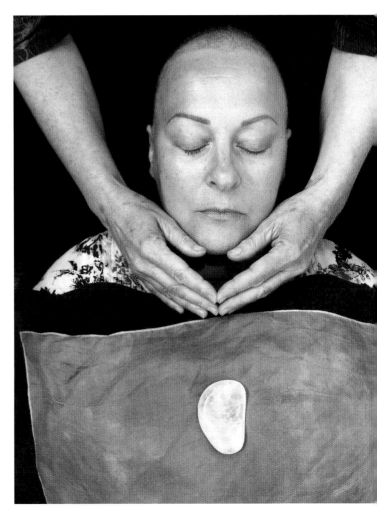

Chakra Balancing with Sarah Fairy. A lovely healing.

Very floaty. The only thing out of balance is my solar plexus. Clearly being bald is not helping my self confidence yet.

Poole Hospital

20 May 2014

"When you are at the mercy of your body and medicine, it is all about control."

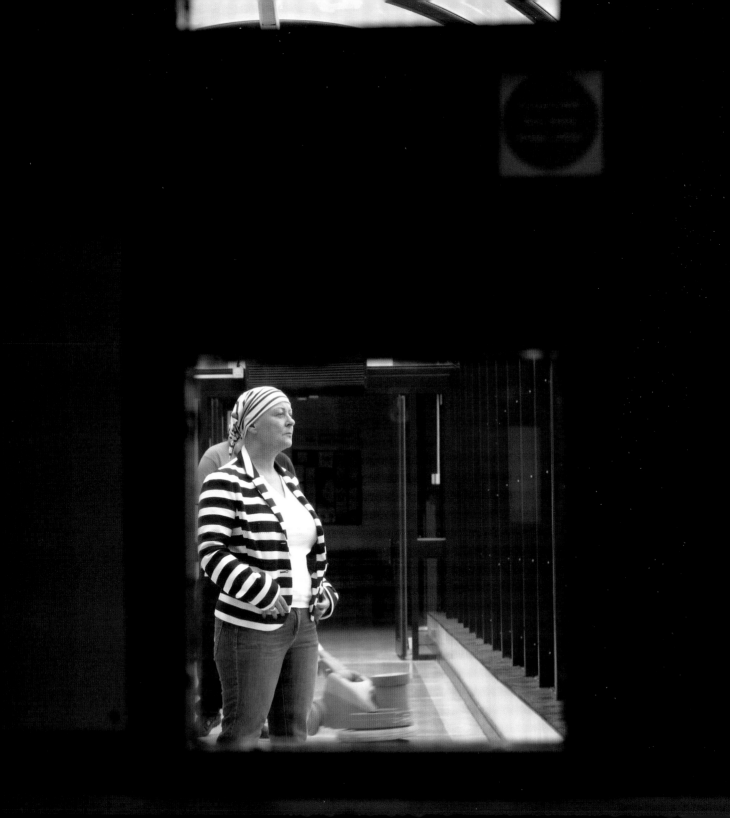

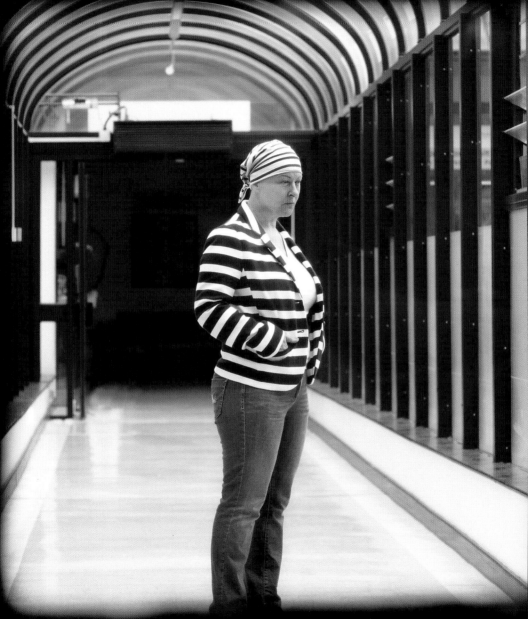

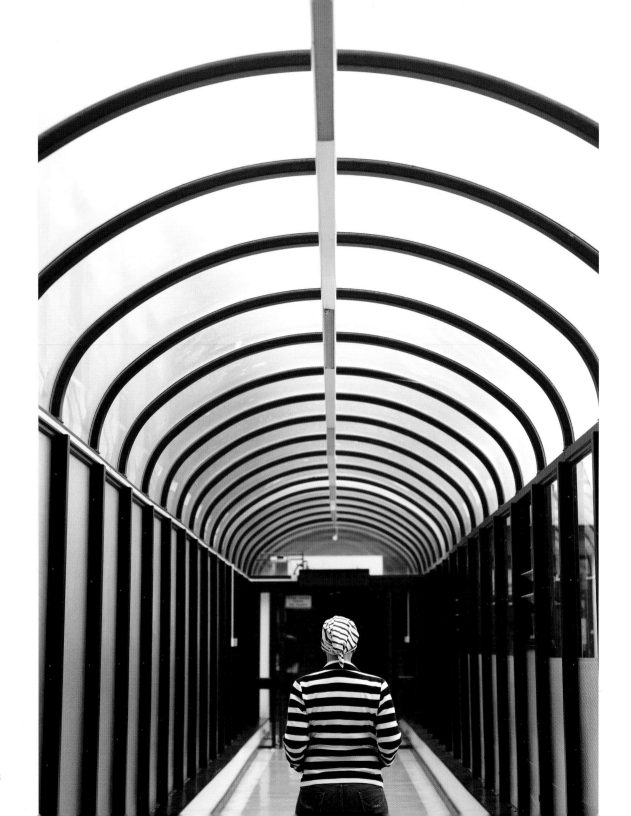

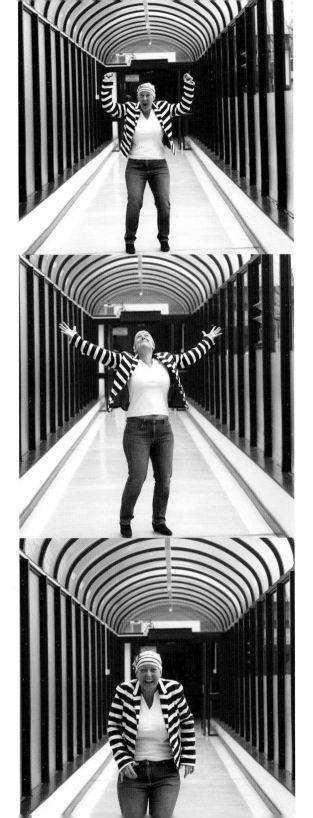

It was quite shocking to go to Poole Hospital for my first appointment. I have felt so safe and known at Salisbury. Suddenly I was in a new bigger environment. I felt anonymous. The architecture was depressing. The cancer unit subterranean.

In the radiotherapy department I was put on a scanner so they could work out the zapping area. It's the whole of the right breast. I was surprised. Somehow I had assumed it would just be the tumour area. Tattoos – considerably more discrete and less painful than my eyebrows - were put at key marker points in my cleavage and flank.

But when I asked about scheduling the dates I was told I had to return for another meeting next week. I expressed how annoyed I was at having to do yet another 3 hour round trip. I have been trying to get dates out of them for weeks. I need to know when I begin and end. It is a huge commitment – every day for three weeks. I need to plan. I felt angry at the scant regard that is given to the huge impact this commitment has on our lives. At a time like this, when you are at the mercy of your body and medicine, it is all about control.

"Hello

It's me again. And another round robin I'm afraid.

Yes, whether you wanted it or not, there has been another request, so here is the latest update. And a new photo too. GI Jane - move over. (Can I add that while Johnnie took a great photo my head is not that lumpy. Indeed my head shape has been massively and gratifyingly admired. Nice.)

Anyway, last week I had my fourth and final chemo. YEAY! That I actually got that far is quite an accomplishment as after the 2nd one I went a little crazy. Indeed, I learnt for the first time that I really do have the capacity to become totally unhinged.

We all know the physical side effects are bad. But so are the mental ones. I became genuinely obsessed that the chemo was doing me more harm than good. So I ended up crying and shouting at the oncologist telling her exactly this. I also added for good measure "I don't care if I die before I'm 65. I'm not having any more fucking chemo." To her credit, she listened calmly and then told me the problem was about me not being in control. She said if I wanted to stop I could, but while I was so distressed she could not let me make that call.

She saw me a week later, by which time I had calmed down having discovered the most brilliant homeopath in Shaftesbury. She spent two hours peeling away my layers and discovering my fears. She acknowledged that my hatred of chemo goes right to the very core of my being. To have chemo is as big a challenge as I could set myself. It is my equivalent of running the London marathon or climbing Everest. I realised that meant I could not stop. If I gave up I would be a failure – and would fail at everything else I ever try in life. Conversely, if I succeeded, then I would be able to succeed in anything I do in future. It became that simple.

Thus, while I stayed convinced that the red poison was not doing me any good, the mental achievement became paramount. Happily the homeopathic remedy was sensationally effective. Despite feeling unbelievably fatigued, I never once became hysterical again. Reluctantly the homeopath had to tell me what I was taking as the oncologist became worried about my liver last week. I have been taking python venom. My other great fear is snakes. So that's what she used. She has attacked one of my deepest fears with the other. Which led to my epiphany – we need to recognise, confront and conquer our fears. Only then are we released to be the person who we truly are.

I do still feel so blessed for the love and support I have received from friends, family and neighbours. Soups, stews, energy bars, almond sate sauce, flowers, body lotions, hats, scarves, a cashmere wrap, a surprise party, dog walking, dog sitting, olive oil (home made in Italy), cards, prayers, meditations, lifts to the hospital... It is just overwhelming. Yesterday when the postman dropped off a card saying he was praying for me and offered to do anything he could I cried (really quite hard) for 15 minutes. The kindness of others. And let me not forget the kindness, the patience, the empathy, and the unswerving love and support from Johnnie. He has had to cop a lot and has never once complained or even turned to drugs (just kidding).

Next stop, daily radiotherapy in Poole for 3 weeks from 9th June. It's a bit of a hike from here, so we are staying in a beach hut/house at Mudeford for some of it. At least that makes it an adventure. And nothing, nothing, will ever be as bad as having chemo.

Thank you to you all for your love and support. If I haven't already told you, I am so blessed to have you in my life.

Love Tiggy xx"

Respite

29 May 2014

"All that stress and worry has lifted. The fear of feeling that weird and sick again has gone"

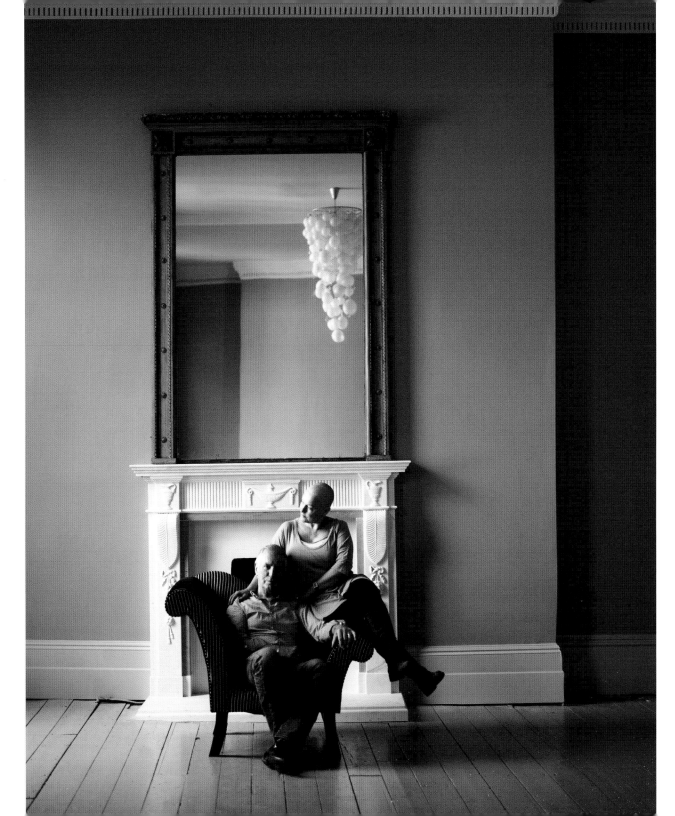

People keep telling me how well I look. I guess because I am jubilant about being through the chemo. All that stress and worry has lifted. The fear of feeling that weird and sick again has gone.

But not just that. I am getting to a place of understanding. The reason I have gone through this is so that I become wiser, so that I understand me better – my health and my spiritual journey.

Bella suggested a photo session with Johnnie at The Grosvenor Arms – Shaftesbury's boutique hotel. I was on a high having just seen Salil for acupuncture. He had just told me how much I have progressed. When he first met me I was angry. Now he says I am not. Indeed, I am not far from the ultimate goal – that is not just to forgive but to feel compassion for those who have hurt you. When you can do that, he says, you have arrived.

Here are his bits of wisdom. In no particular order.

1. If you don't take a rest, the Universe will make you.
2. No health professional can heal you. All they can do is remove the blocks that are stopping you heal yourself. If the body can, it will always move towards balance. If it cannot it is because of the blocks.
3. It is only when you can see the world beyond yourself that suffering ceases.
4. In the current Western world we are all held in the position of a child. For a child the world revolves around them, while a true adult releases that need – they allow the world to just happen and are simply a part of it. Yet so much of the media perpetuates the child in us - soap operas, Jeremy Kyle, the celebrity culture – all encourage the ego and us being the centre of the world.

On a practical level, he has also told me to stop writing lists. I THRIVE on lists. He argues it is me trying to be in control, but it just creates the illusion that I am. They don't make things better. Indeed, they make things worse.
How can he mean that?

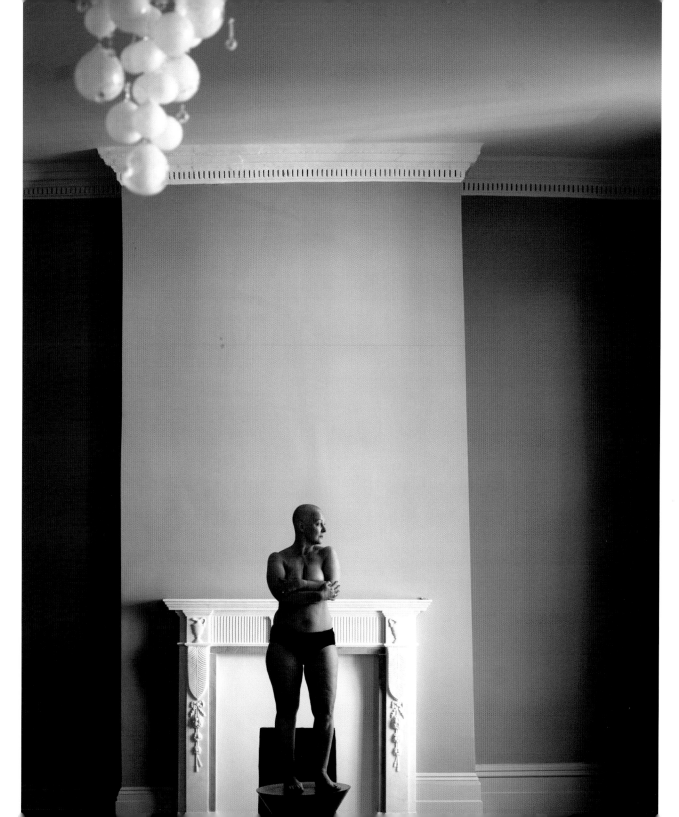

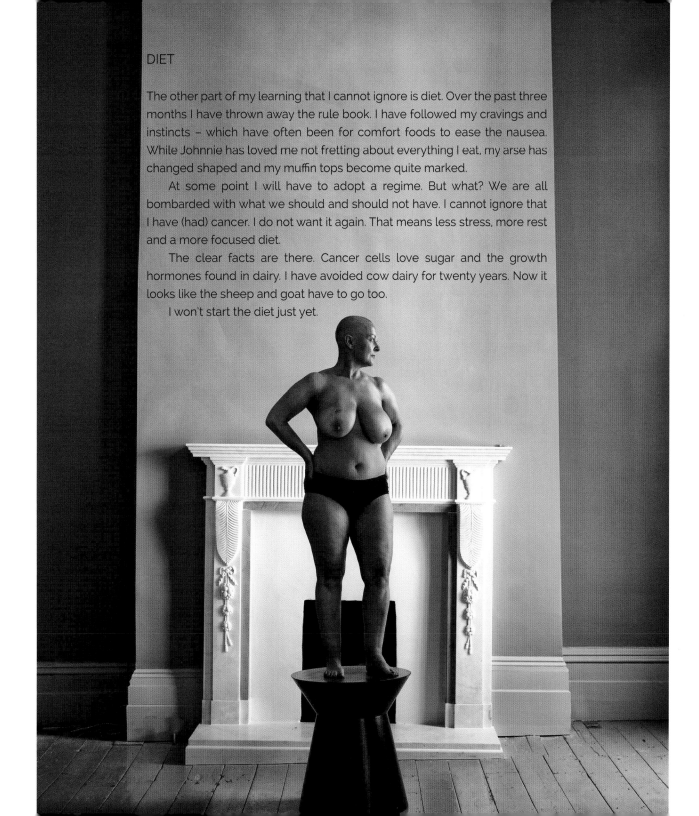

DIET

The other part of my learning that I cannot ignore is diet. Over the past three months I have thrown away the rule book. I have followed my cravings and instincts – which have often been for comfort foods to ease the nausea. While Johnnie has loved me not fretting about everything I eat, my arse has changed shaped and my muffin tops become quite marked.

At some point I will have to adopt a regime. But what? We are all bombarded with what we should and should not have. I cannot ignore that I have (had) cancer. I do not want it again. That means less stress, more rest and a more focused diet.

The clear facts are there. Cancer cells love sugar and the growth hormones found in dairy. I have avoided cow dairy for twenty years. Now it looks like the sheep and goat have to go too.

I won't start the diet just yet.

Radiotherapy

10 June 2014

" I was about to start the next challenge on the
cancer assault course and neither J nor I had
prepared for it"

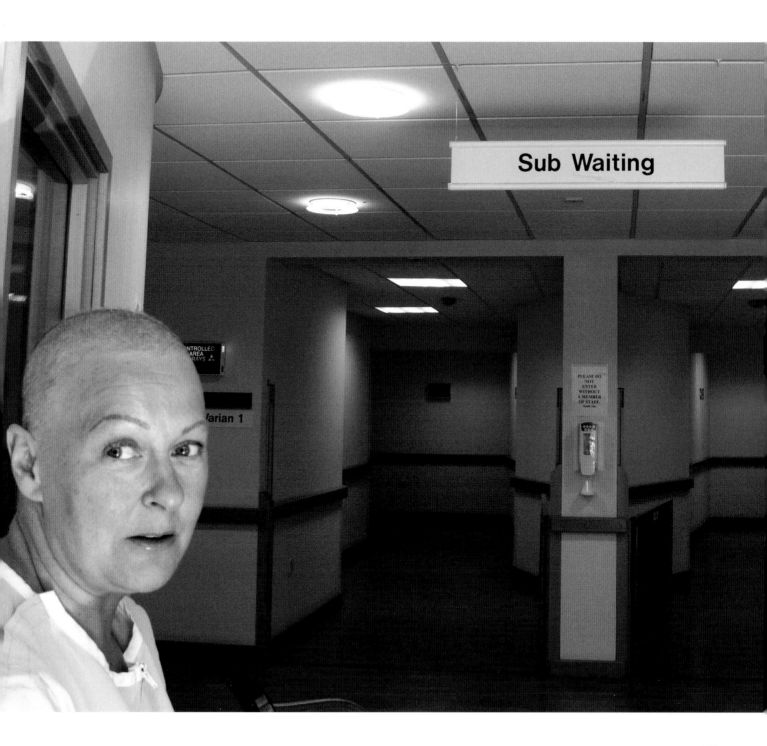

Sub Waiting

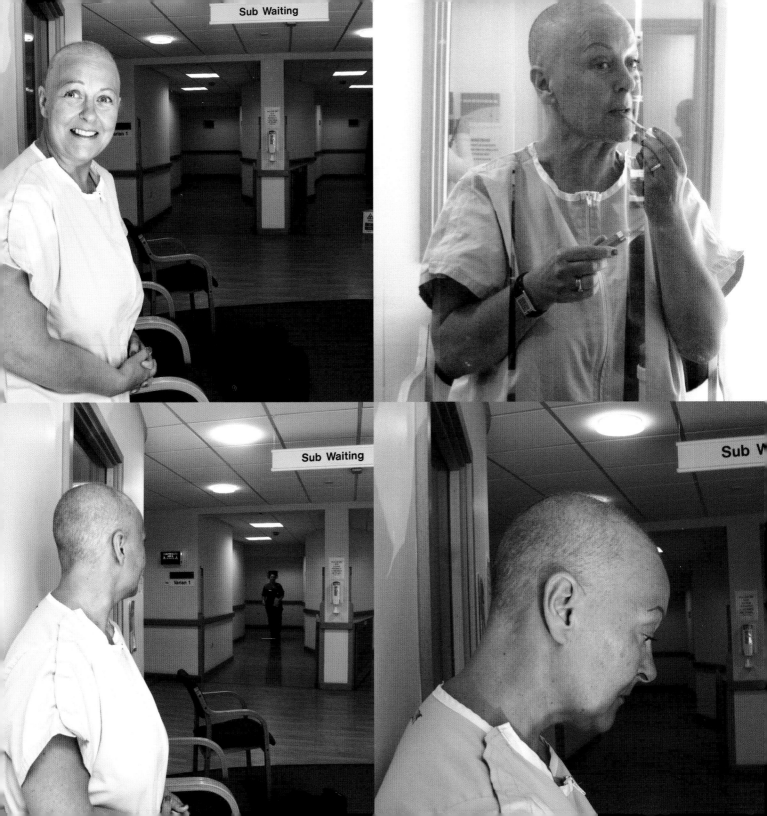

The calm after the storm. I am sat on the steps of our friend Sarah's beach hut no. 178 at Mudeford Spit. The sun is blasting down on me. On us – as Johnnie and Darcey are at the bottom of the step. The sea is gently rolling in and the Isle of White and its Needles sit on the horizon.

And thank God for this beautiful summer's day – for yesterday there was a storm. Not outside but within me and with Johnnie, who was inevitably pulled in to my drama.

Yesterday I went to Poole Hospital for the first of 15 radiotherapy sessions. I had not prepared for it in any way. The weekend had been 'as normal' with various social events including Johnnie opening the Shaftesbury Festival and attending a cream tea and service in a barn in aid of Milton on Stour's church spire. As you do. As we do.

But as we drove to the hospital I started to cry. To sob in fact. Because it hit me. Life is NOT 'as normal'. I was about to start the next challenge on the cancer assault course and neither J nor I had prepared for it. Indeed I feel that J has forgotten I am even having treatment still. We have slipped back to the usual way of me doing everything – helped enormously by his new Triumph Thunderbird motorbike and the good weather – every possible chance he is off.

Added to this, on Sunday, I started taking homeopathic python venom again to support me through the radio.

What happened took us both by surprise. As the journey progressed I cried more and more. Anger welled up in me. Not fierce, but a gentle anger. I guess from fear. But I had to tell Johnnie what was in my head.

If it hadn't been for our marriage I felt I would not now have cancer. I was not attacking but merely airing. A decade of dramas and upset. Things I've had to suppress and absorb.

I said it was part of my healing to let this out. To expel all thoughts and energies that may be blocking me as I do not want the cancer to return.

It did not make for an easy day. Johnnie dropped me at the hospital door and drove off. I was in tears when I met the radiographer. I told her it was nerves.

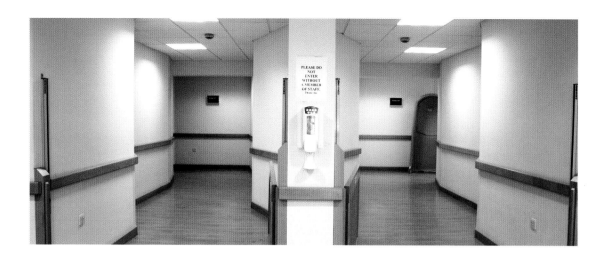

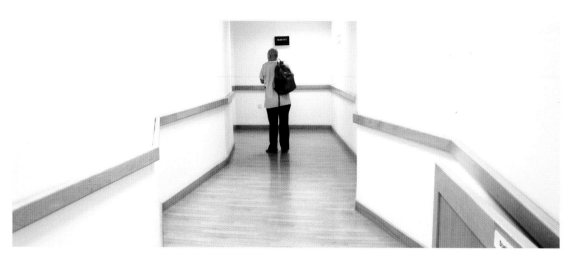

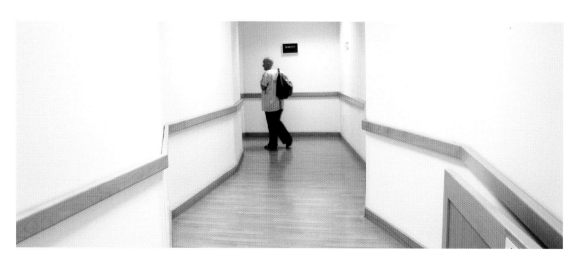

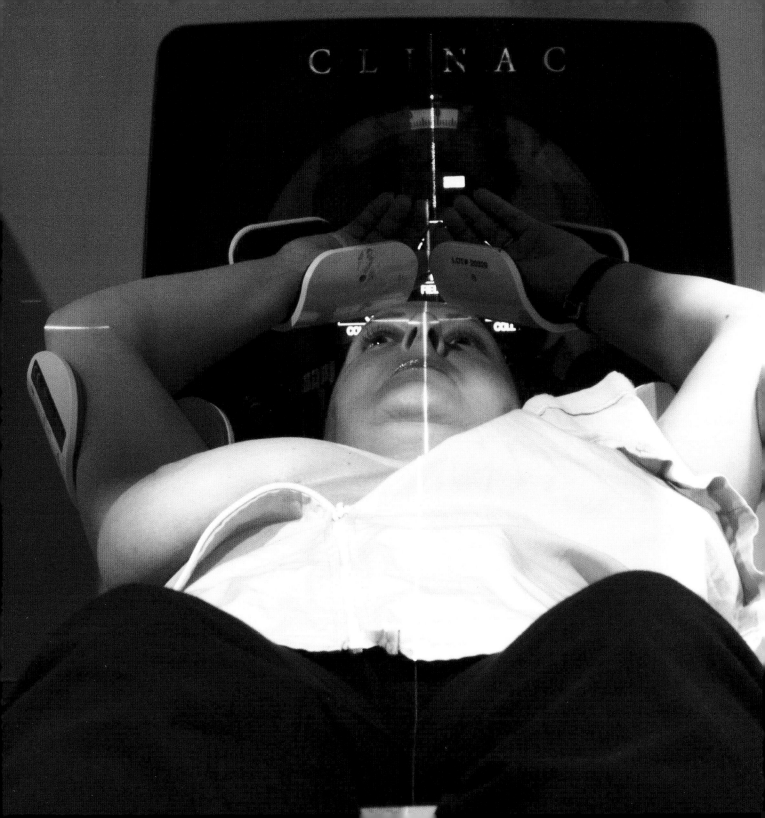

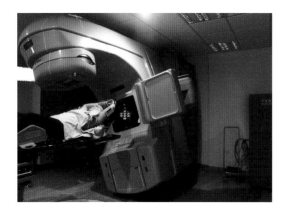
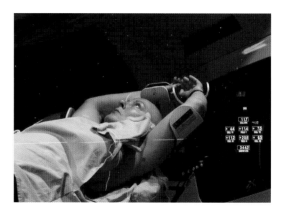
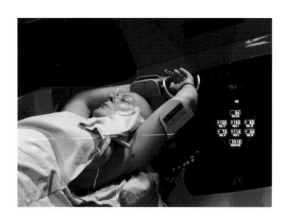
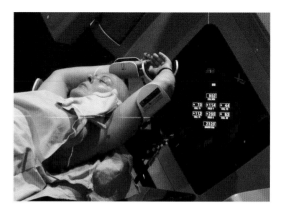

The session was fascinating. Much time was spent lining up my tattoos with green lines of marker light. The arm of the extraordinary and huge Varian machine moved around me to zap me in different positions. I had to lie still. No room for tears or a heaving chest here. When the radiation is given the machine makes a noticeable tone for about twenty seconds in each position. The room is dark. You are alone. You feel like an extra in Star Trek. Where might I beam up to?

Afterwards I felt knocked about. I was nauseous, tired and headachy. 'Oh Christ' I thought. Three weeks of this? I can't bare it.

Johnnie came and found me. There was a truce. With great effort we got ourselves to the beach hut from Hengistbury Head via the 'Noddy Train'. (Only in England would such a dramatic day involve riding a toy train.)

As the evening descended there were more words, more tears. Finally we fell in to each others' arms, professed our love and exhausted went to bed as the sun went down.

While yesterday Johnnie felt the marriage could not survive, today we have woken refreshed to this beautiful day. I slept for 12 hours. As well as I have in months. The lack of WIFI, noise, electricity, light and the gentle sea air enabled me to have the most healing sleep.

Now we have to set off for session 2. I am not nervous today. I know what is in store. The only thing I dread is the roomful of moaning men in the waiting area because the machines are running late. We're lucky to be using them for free aren't we?

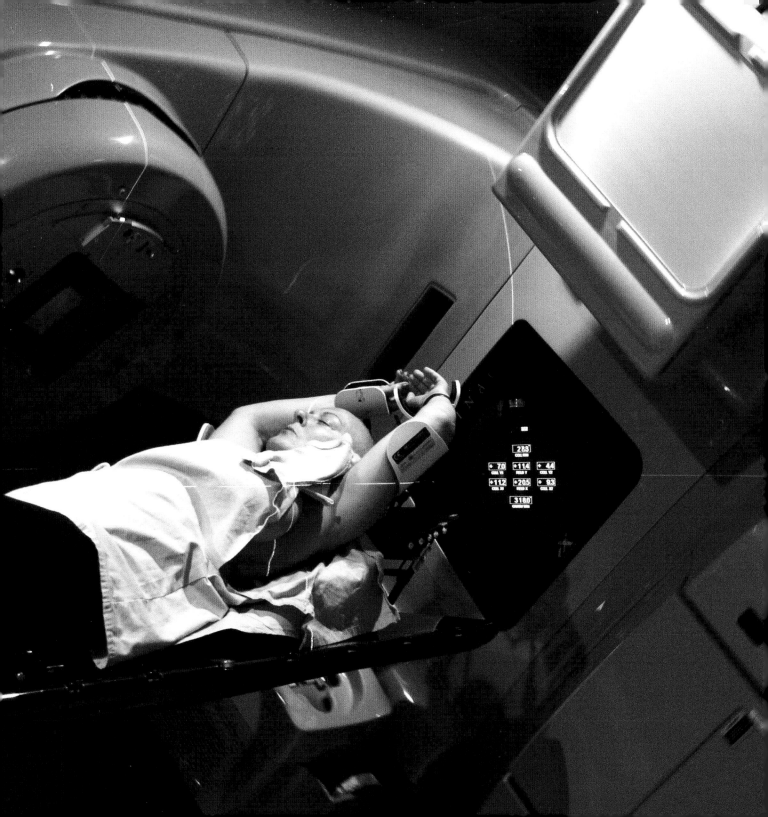

Hut 178

10 June 2014

" At one stage hats and scarves were coming at me from every angle. And I have thoroughly loved wearing them."

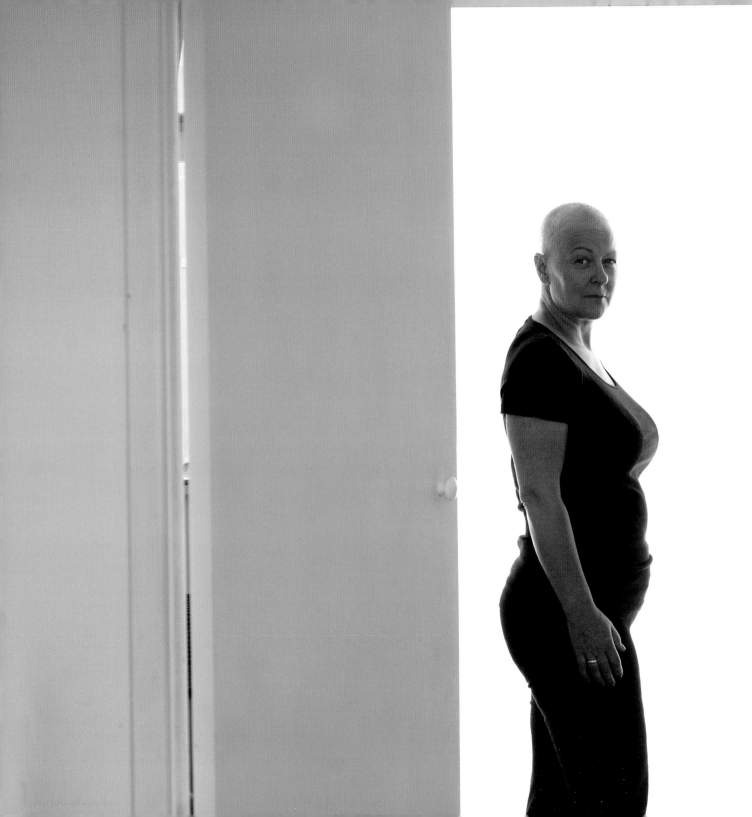

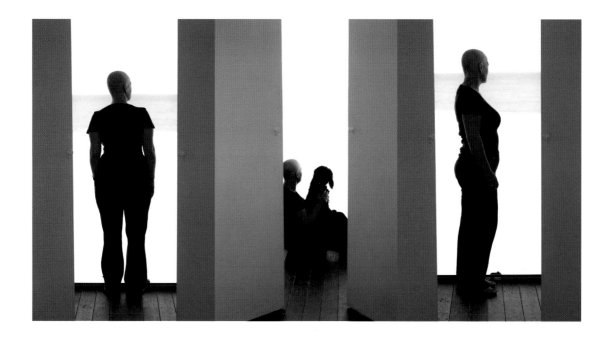

Bella joined me today to capture the joy that is radiotherapy. Afterwards she came to the beach hut for our 'hat shoot'. We have planned this for a while. My oldest girlfriend Anneke sent a new hat after each chemo. It has been a source of great hilarity as she became more and more extreme in her choices. Then there were the knitted ones that 90 year old Mrs Tolfrey made me. At one stage hats and scarves were coming at me from every angle. And I have thoroughly loved wearing them.

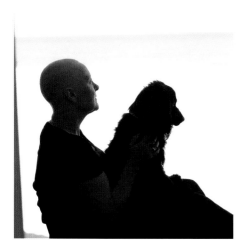
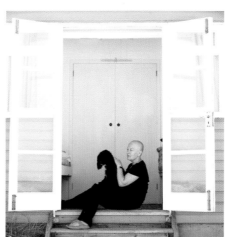
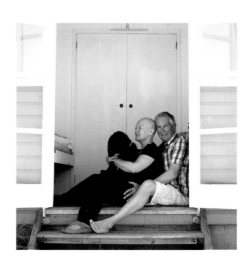

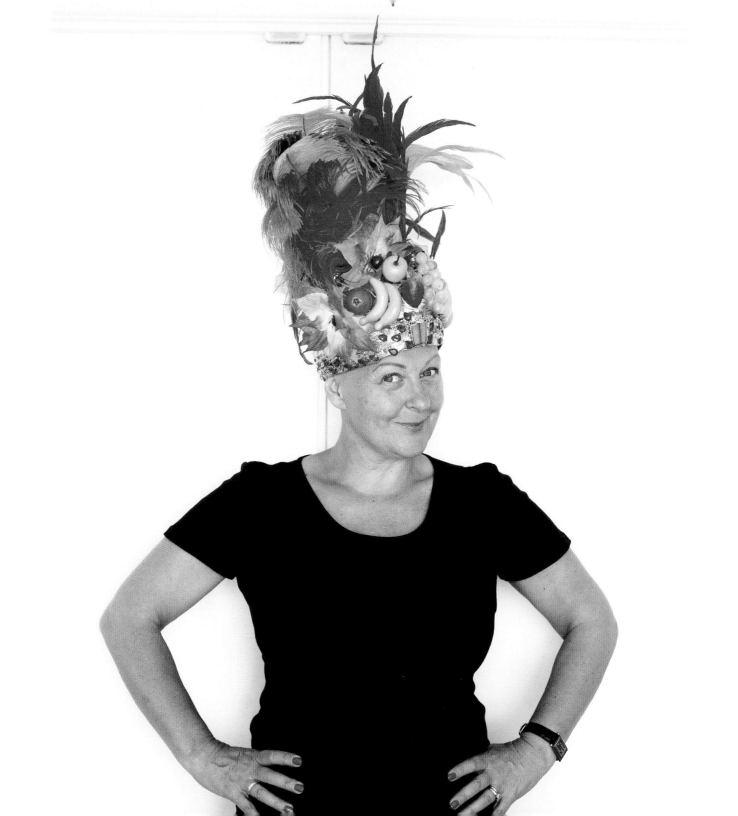

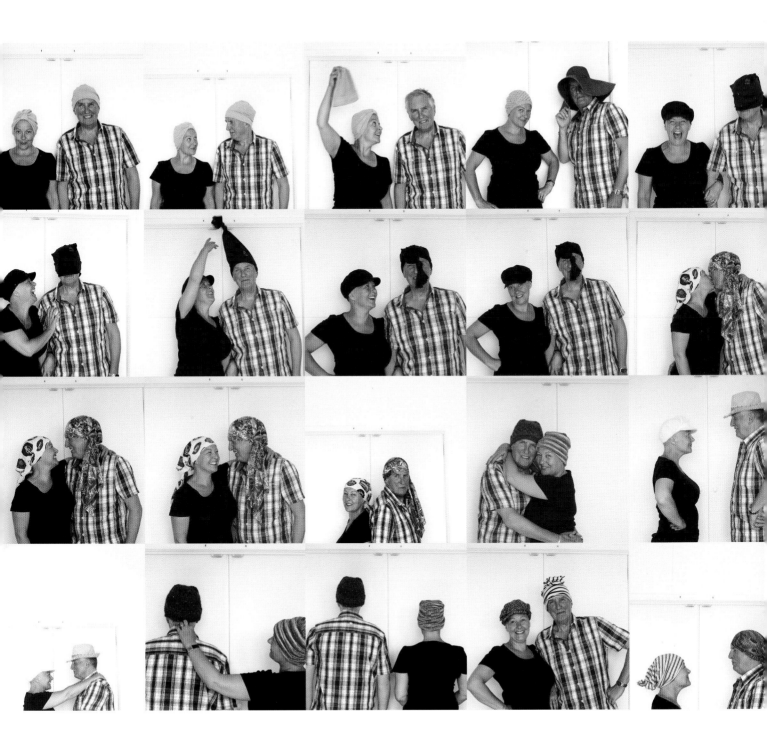

18 June 2014

Back in the beach hut - alone. I've slept a glorious 11 hours. I hadn't realised how tired I am. Perhaps I should have been taking naps after each radio session.

Things have gone rat shit with J again. Why? Perhaps the pressure of daily treatments and needing to be taken, perhaps the deprivation of sugar and carbs from the diet as I try to detox, or perhaps it is something more sinister.

Since the first day of radio I have felt surges of anger towards him. Yesterday afternoon we had a fight about someone who wants to borrow our London flat. It was horrible. I don't really have the energy to argue and asked him to stop. But there is anger in him too. Pent up emotion.

Without doubt the stress of my situation and driving me daily is getting to him. I don't blame him. I remember driving 28 days on the trot when he was in Salisbury hospital (while also doing a house move). With his endless requests I became exhausted.

He stormed out yesterday and took the dog. I turned off my phone. Since then I have been gloriously alone. Just me and the sea. It is so healing. Everything in life is rushed today. With constant interruptions. Here it is slow – and there is no one to bother me.

Right now I feel smothered, beholden, and not in my power. Johnnie is well known, well loved, in demand. His energy field is large. It has been bloody hard to be in my power since I have met him.

We normally have a couple of days apart each week when one of us is in London. With this bloody treatment that is not happening and I am feeling a huge resentment. I hate not being independent and self sufficient. I am really bored of all this treatment. And Herceptin looms - a year of it.

19 June 2014

He came back. After writing the above I slept and slept. The sea ahead of me. Phone off. Silence… Until Johnnie knocked on the door scaring the wits out of me.

The rings are back on. We have kissed and made up. We have enjoyed the glorious weather and swam in the sea.

Sadly we have packed up and left the beach hut. No more early morning walks and yoga on Hengistbury Head, no more listening to the sea at night, and no more Noddy Train. But Hut 178 did its job. It was healing. And it gave me the space to explain to Johnnie I need to get my power back.

I'm now waiting for my blast. Varian 2 is running 40 minutes late today. The waiting area becomes quite sociable. You see the same faces each day. Mainly men having prostate cancer treatment. Seven weeks of it, poor bastards.

When people have finished their course they leave a celebratory box of chocolates. A lot of people have finished today – we have two boxes of Thornton's Premium, a box of Celebrations (just too obvious) and some Chocolate Orange 'Segsations'. A new one on me. I am resisting them all. I am off sugar, wheat and dairy. Anything to reduce the muffin top and arse.

But here is today's dilemma. When I finish what should I leave? Sugar feeds cancer. If there is only one thing you should quit it is that. A point that the majority of cancer specialists and their patients ignore.

24 June 2014

Since reading up the side effects of Herceptin I have been worried. Being me I wanted to back out of it. So Poole Hospital got me an appointment with one of their oncologists today. He told me that it is the single most valuable post operative treatment I can have. This he says with just 3 more radioactive blasts to go.

I left the hospital feeling weak. It's going on and on. I wobbled as I climbed the stairs to the outside world. Back home I couldn't stay awake. Not even through Andy Murray's opening match at Wimbledon. They warned me that the fatigue would set in this week. And so it has. I feel as if I've hit a brick wall.

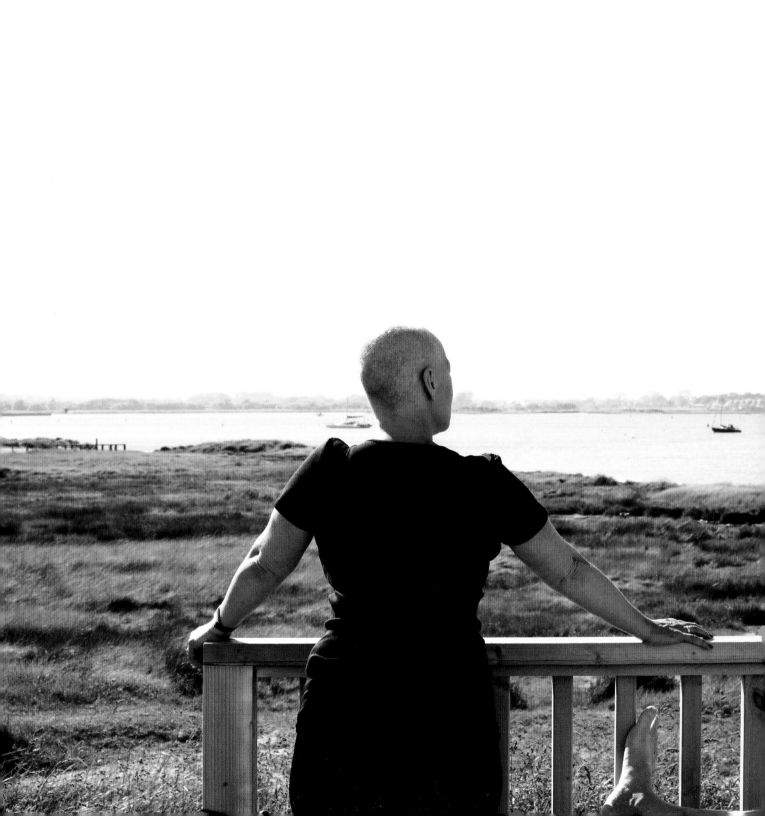

Final Radiotherapy

27 June 2014

" Each day my waking thought has been whether I have radiotherapy that day."

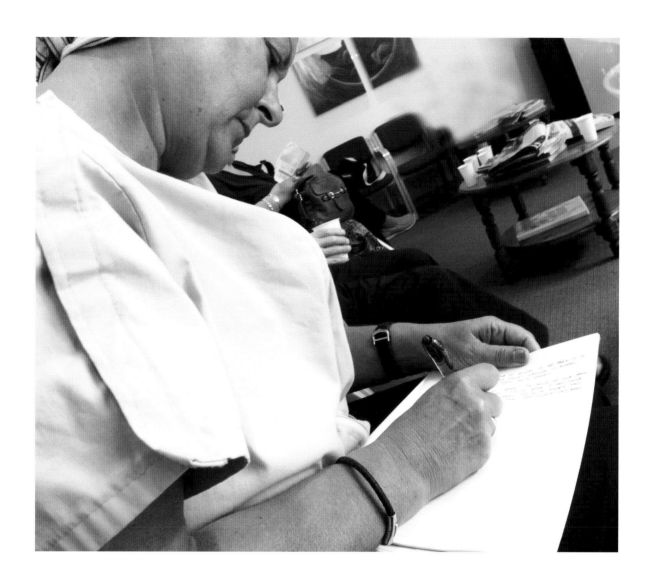

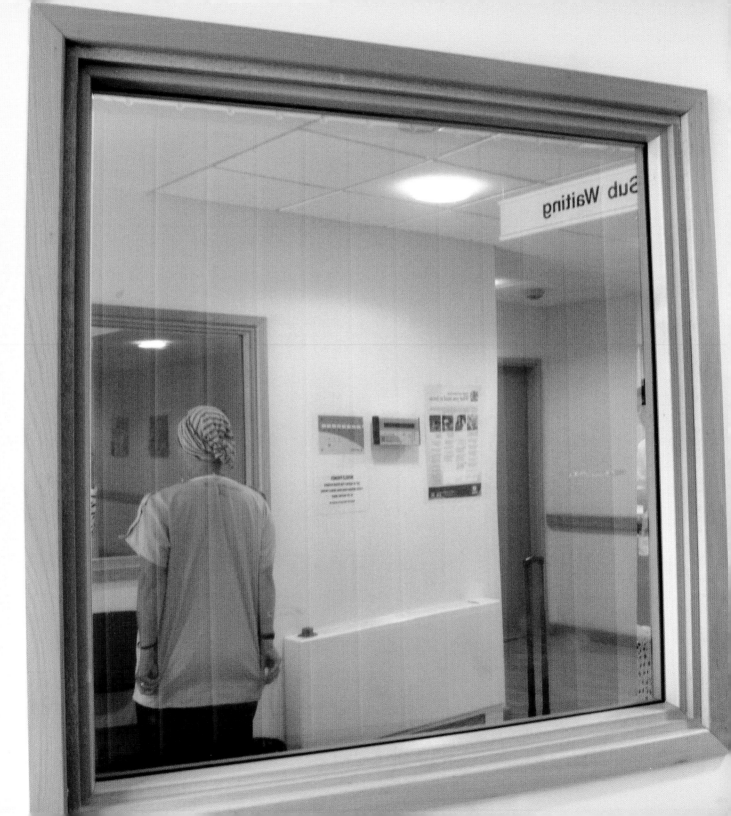

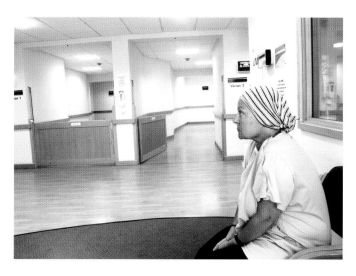
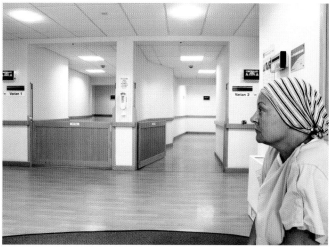
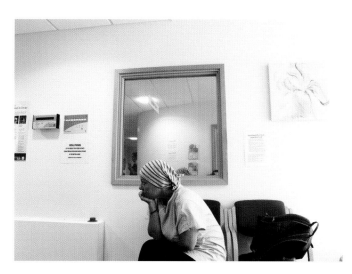
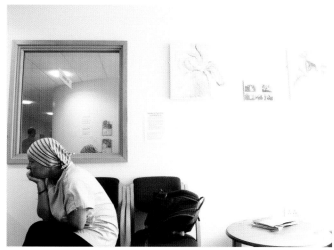

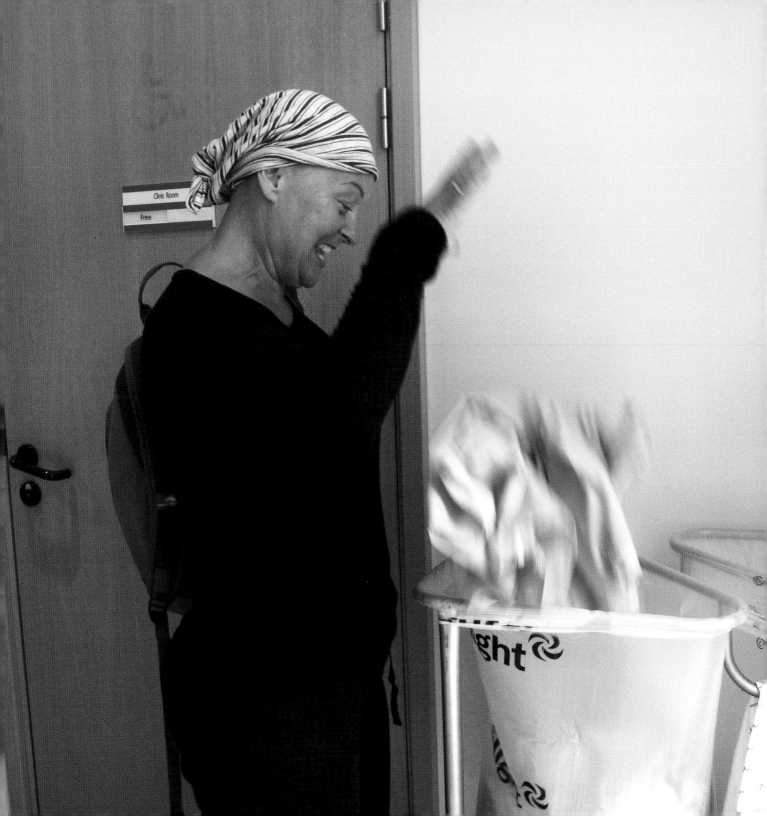

27 June 2014

My final radio day. And to finish off the experience there is a huge delay on the Varian machine.

This week has been an effort. I got quite depressed mid week. I wanted to run away from everyone and everything. The drive alone has taken its toll. It's a good three hour round trip. Each day my waking thought has been whether I have radiotherapy that day. The answer has been a consistent 'yes'.

The radiographers have been lovely. I got so relaxed in front of them that one day this week I walked in and mistakenly took off my lilac gown and stood there breasts out. We were all embarrassed. Me most. Even though they expose my breast each day, there is a huge line between standing there – fulsome brazen breasts hanging – and lying on the bed where they are the object of the treatment.

What a very definite full stop to these three weeks it was to throw away the lilac gown. Another stage is complete. Another box ticked.

(PS. I didn't leave chocolates. I am ashamed to say I left nothing.)

28 June 2014

It's not just the hair on my head growing back. I feel like an adolescent again. It means a return to normality. Although not having to worry about depilation has been a positive advantage.

30 June 2014

Back at Salisbury Hospital. A cause for celebration. So lovely to be back where everyone knows your name.

I saw Claire my oncologist who, all of a sudden, is very pregnant. Naturally I voiced my desire not to have Herceptin. She made a strong case for it, and said she had not taken the decision lightly. She also said a year would be better than six months. I did not want to hear that.

As it was the first jab – a slowly administered five-minute injection into the leg – I had to lie there for six hours in case I had a reaction. It was delightful to lie still, so quietly. I brought my post and laptop. I got through masses of the relentless admin and pestering emails that invade our lives.

The only thing I didn't like – hearing the 'bing bong' of the chemo drips when they are empty. The sound brings back horrific memories of feeling sick.

1 July 2014

I can't quite believe it. A treatment without a ghastly side effect.

Thank the Lord.

Radiation Damage

3 July 2014

" I am not sure if it was the size of my breasts or the uniquely positioned burn, but she had never seen anything like it."

Oh my God. My breast looks as if it has leprosy. I took off my sports bra after some self imposed 'let's get the body back' exercise, and as it came off so did an eight inch layer of of skin from under my breast. So sore.

I went to see a nurse at the surgery. I am not sure if it was the size of my breasts or the uniquely positioned burn, but she had never seen anything like it. Even the skin around my nipple is coming off. Gross.

Sonya, the lovely breast care nurse, has arranged for me to go to the burns unit on Monday.

7 July 2014

Johnnie warned me I wasn't up to it and he was right. A weekend on the Isle of White with the 'Inner Sanctum' gang of friends was not the recuperative joy I had imagined it would be. I simply could not cope and lost it.

Virginia sat with me in the bathroom as I sobbed baring my sore breast. I thought the whole thing would come off, the nipple at the very least.

The burns unit nurse today assured me that I would be retaining the whole breast and sent me away with plenty of suitably shaped dressings. I have been worried about getting an infection. Sometimes all you need is a bit of reassurance to make you feel better.

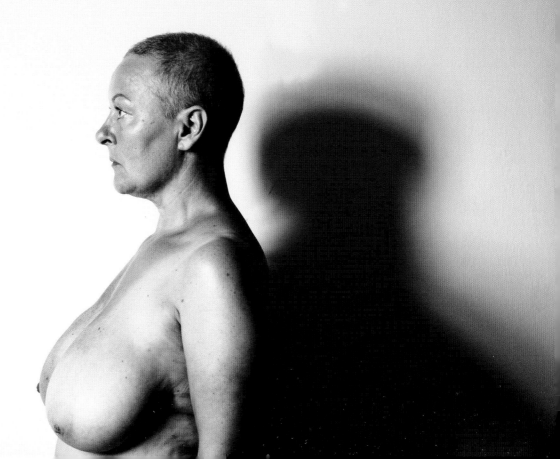

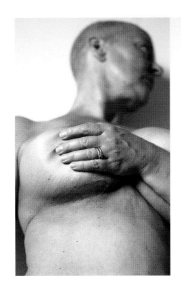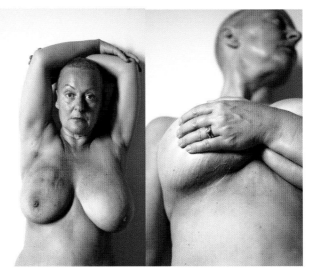

9 July 2014

A cheap day return to London. I woke intimidated by the day ahead afraid of the train, the crowds, the getting around.

I had an appointment with Tony Monkcom, my alternative doctor who prescribes my vitamins and minerals. It was good to see him, even though I cried.

And afterwards to go to Itsu again. Who ever thought that a salmon salad could be such a high in someone's life?

Then the treat of the Matisse Cut-Outs at Tate Modern. The story of a man, in his eighties, reinventing himself with the help of a rather beautiful assistant. I returned home exhausted but inspired.

14 August 2014

Our friends Frank and Rozzi have leant us their beautiful house "Bobola" on Paxos. It is so healing to be here, perched up on a hill looking out over Loggos harbour.

But we only just got here. Just before we went to the Gate at Gatwick I realised I did not have my passport. I had left it in security.

I howled into Johnnie's chest that we would have to miss the flight. I have become so stupid, so careless. The capable producer has become a liability.

Thank God for the man who found it. I wouldn't miss being here. And I am glad to be out of the UK today. The Mail ran an article about us being the new Patrons of Carers UK. I don't mind getting publicity but I am always nervous to read it.

Manor Farm

22 August 2014

" The house is starting to take shape.
It feels as if my life is too."

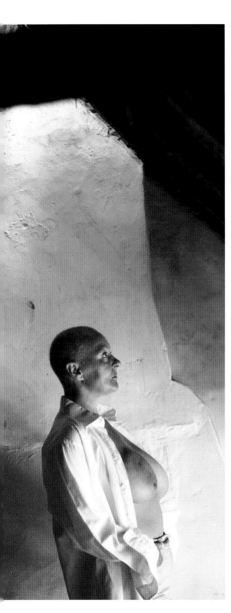

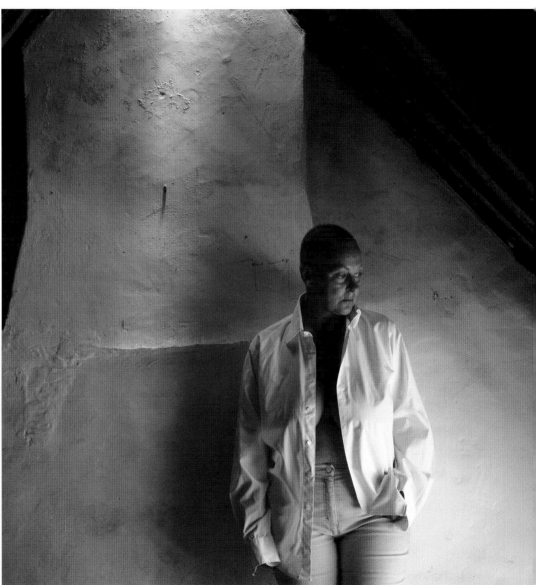

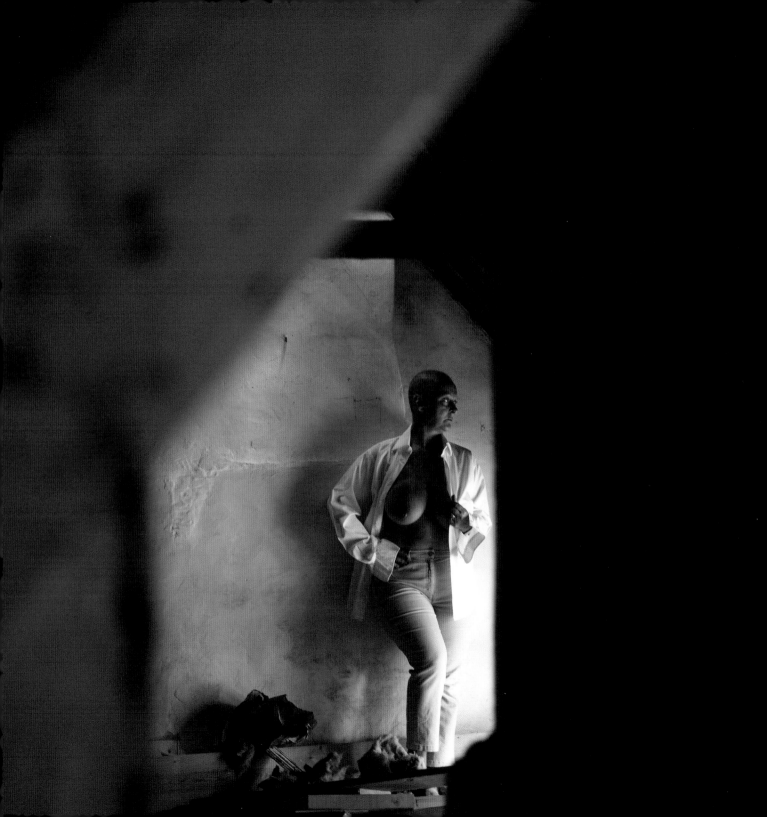

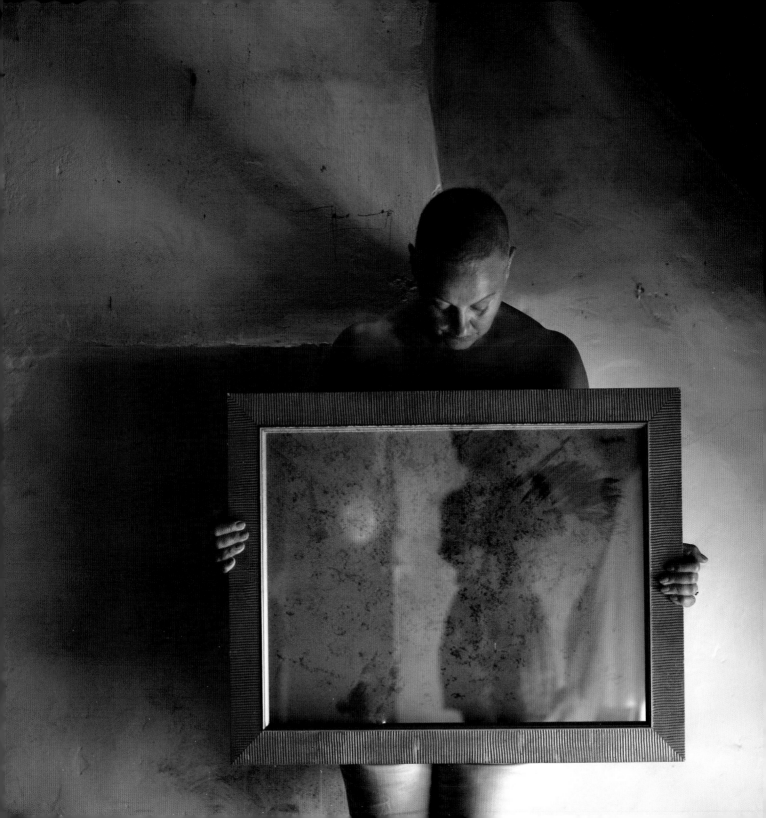

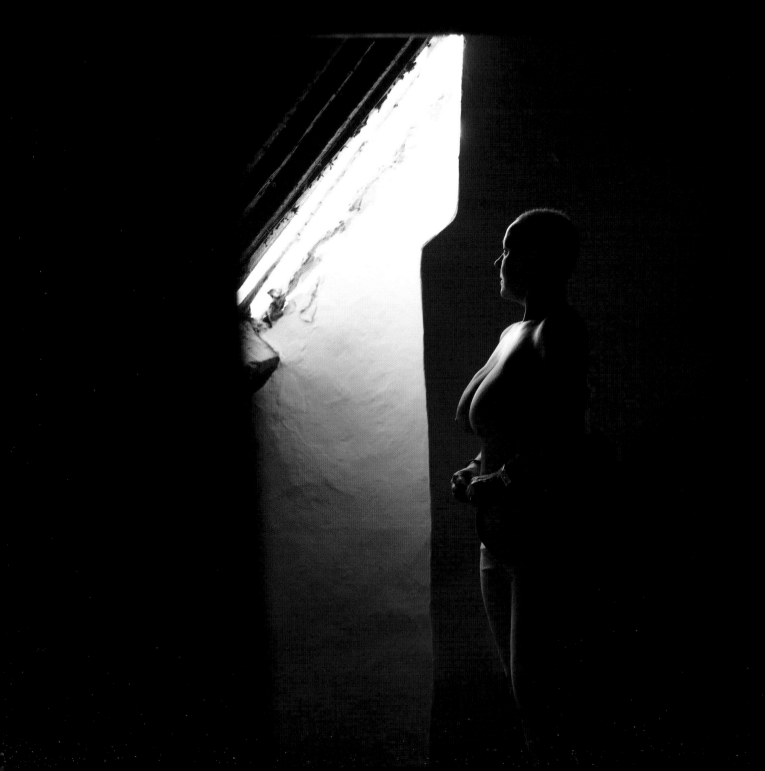

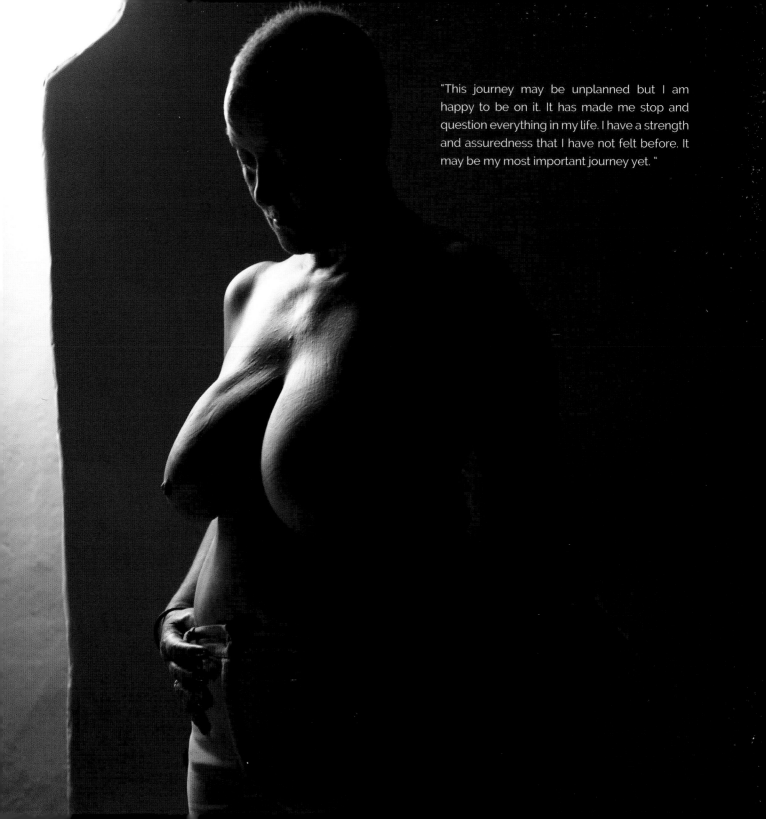

"This journey may be unplanned but I am happy to be on it. It has made me stop and question everything in my life. I have a strength and assuredness that I have not felt before. It may be my most important journey yet. "

"Hello

I thought I should bring the round robins to an end and let you all know that I am fine. Indeed, I am well. Too much going on – but hey, who hasn't.

Radiotherapy in June was boring and tiring, but without it we wouldn't have had a fantastic time staying in a beach hut at Mudeford Spit. The simplicity of life was fabulous, the sun hot and the sea healing. The radiotherapy firmed the boob up beautifully which was a bonus, although the apparent leprosy as it burned and peeled was not.

It's an ill wind that blows no good and one result of my little ordeal is that the charity, Carers UK have asked Johnnie and I to be their joint patrons. Next year is their 50th anniversary so we will be involved in a number of events to help raise awareness and money. You may want to be very wary of my emails in future. I am bound to be asking you a favour.

To help publicise Carers UK we did an interview with Rebecca Hardy at The Mail. She did an article on us ten years ago when Johnnie returned to work after his cancer. The main thing I took from the article is that I am now much fatter with cropped hair. Charming. As they showed photos of me ten years ago I didn't think it needed to be said. But the weight and short hair are inevitable factors of breast cancer. Sad but true. I am actually rather liking my Dame Judy hair styling. I may keep it that way. I hope to shed the pounds. The article is somewhat melodramatic. They certainly know how to edit a sentence. When I read it I thought 'oh dear God – I'm not going to make it'

While my energy and fitness both have a long way to go (and it would seem, my weight) it is fabulous to feel like a normal person again. Tomorrow I am going to a caravan in Cornwall alone to write for a week. 'Antonia' is making a come back. It has been healthy to step away from her and now great to return. I've been doing some unbelievable coaching with my friend Karin. She has been helping me obliterate any negatives or insecurities I have been harbouring. There were plenty.

I still have Herceptin jabs every three weeks. They tire me for a few days, probably as it affects the heart. And keeps me fat. Also my brain is still pretty mushy. I forget or mislay most things. Like my passport at Gatwick. But most things return. Like the passport. I hope my previous clarity and quick thinking will too.

Anyway – this is my final group thank you to you all.

I am so glad I've had this episode. It has been the most fabulous punctuation mark. I anticipate my life PC being very much more rewarding, wise and under control than it was BC. I could almost recommend it.

Love as always.
Tiggy xx

Ps. Building works on Manor Farm House continue. We should be in before Christmas."

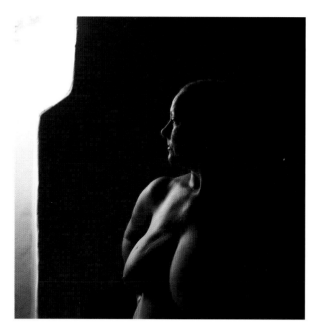
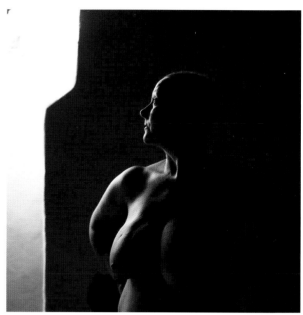
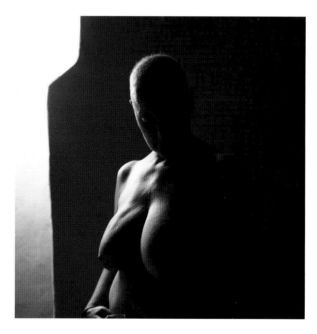
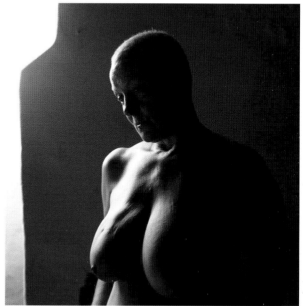

Echogram/Herceptin

11 September 2014

" I was convinced I would be signed off today.
No such luck. My heart is fine. I am fine."

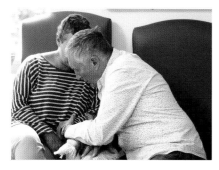
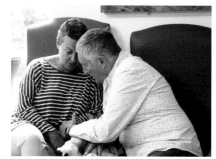
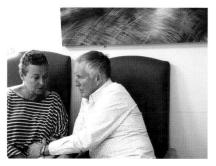
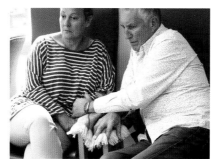
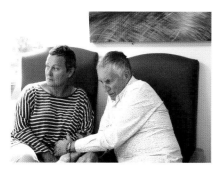
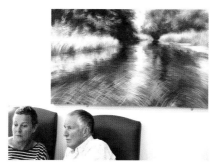
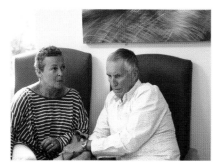
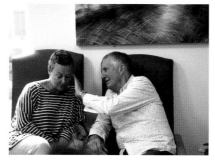

Am I a hypochondriac? Or am I just desperate for any excuse to stop having treatment? Today I had an echocardiogram and ECG. One of the worst side effects of Herceptin is that it can weaken your heart wall. Needless to say I have convinced myself that this is happening to me, particularly due to my heaving chest and shortness of breath whenever I exercise (I have now given up exercising). My mind went into overdrive and I started worrying that the stab of pain I felt was the start of a heart attack. I was convinced I would be signed off today. No such luck. My heart is fine. I am fine. You would think I should be pleased. But it meant I had to have Herceptin 4.

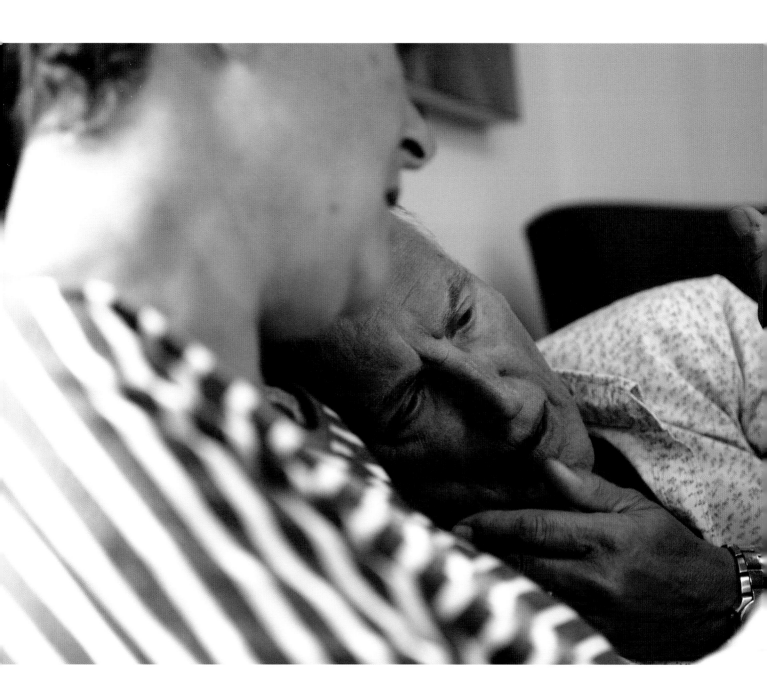

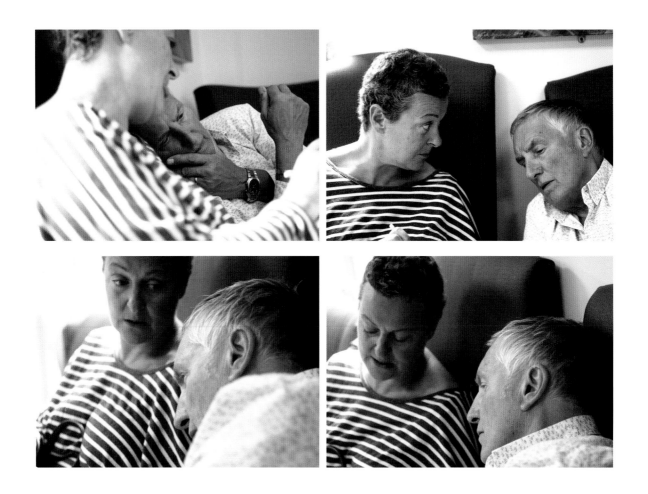

16 October 2014

A CT scan on my BRAIN. I mentioned at my last clinic that I'd had a fit on holiday. I had fallen on a boat badly twisting my ankle. The pain was extreme. I thought it had broken. I passed out and apparently contorted my entire body and face for over 20 seconds. Johnnie thought I was dying. And possibly I was as I did see the most amazing rapid moving multi coloured scenes ending with me facing a man in his 30's. I don't know who he was but I did not want to leave him. Maybe he was Jesus. Johnnie sat next to me as my hands tried to cling on to this other world. "Don't go Tigs" he repeated. Against my will, he pulled me back.

 I don't think for one moment I have a brain tumour. But I do think I had a near death experience and from that I would say that there is certainly a vividly coloured existence that awaits us all.

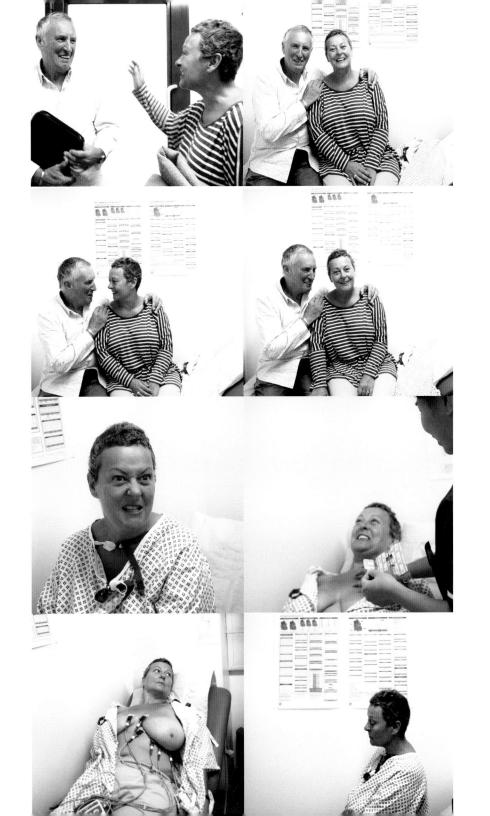

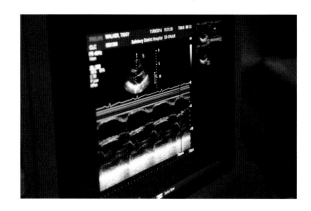

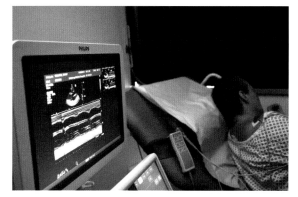

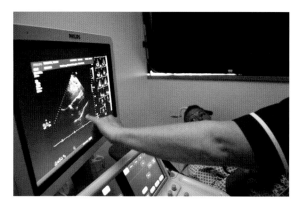

31 October 2014

Back to Joe the personal trainer today. I shared a class with Gary who has broken his collar bone in a bike accident.

What a pair.

I have shied away from exercise as my strength has been so low. And it shows. I stared at my increased stomach in the mirror. It's no longer a muffin top. It's an entire box of muffins. When I bent over to touch my toes I could feel a tyre had formed around my midriff. And that despite the fact that we haven't drunk any booze through October. I should be slimmer. I defensively told Joe it was due to Herceptin affecting my metabolism. I'm not sure he believed me. I'm not sure I did.

3 November 2014

In many ways this is one of the most vulnerable times. The nasty treatments are done. The herceptin jabs are every three weeks – just to keep me in the patient role. But otherwise life returns to normal. Except that it shouldn't. I have been more exhausted – utterly spent – in the last two weeks than I have all year.

Last week Salil was struck by my complete lack of energy. He said I was being kept going by anger alone. His needles were going to release that, and the result was as he predicted. I couldn't function. Could hardly talk. That evening we had a treat – Ballet Rambert at the Theatre Royal Bath. I loved all three sequences. But in each interval I slept in my seat. People were laughing, talking, drinking, engaging. And then there was me. Insular, small, and wondering if I'll ever have the energy to 'live' again.

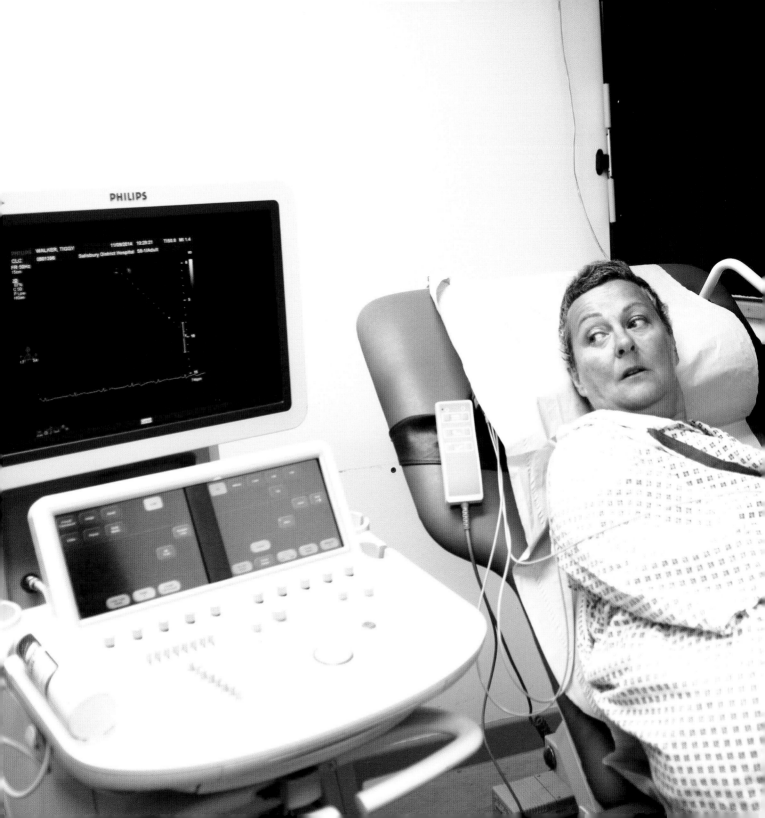

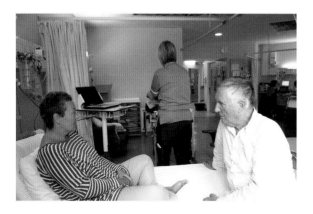

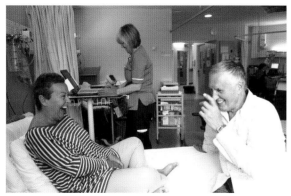

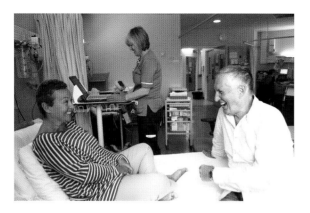

11 November 2014

What the doctors do not know yet, but I do, is that I am going to stop Herceptin at the half way point. Herceptin keeps your blood levels down. The immune system low. The weight up. I know for certain from doctors both Western and Alternative that my kidneys and liver are struggling (despite no drinking).

It may seem mad to others when women fought to get this drug in the first place. But I feel that the huge effect it is having on my energy levels and my complete inability to cope with any stress or difficulty is more likely to make me ill than getting cancer again.

They are doing research with women having it for only six months so they must think it works in this time. I also remember that my oncologist Claire – before we lost her to motherhood – said that because of my liver she might take me off at six months. Thus I do not feel that my act of rebellion is that dangerous or foolhardy.

17 December 2014

"You are clearly beating this." The best words spoken to me all year.

They came from Tony Monkcom, the alternative doctor who measures my levels and immune system with his Vegatest machine. While I am clearly still profoundly tired (correct) he says I am getting stronger and my body is showing it. So the vast array of vitamins I take (about 20 pills a day) and the homeopathy are doing their thing. This positive affirmation, these five words, have given me the biggest boost.

It supports my announcement to the oncologist last week that I am stopping Herceptin on 2nd January. He was understanding and accepting. "As long as you will not regret this decision if it returns". "It won't" was my reply.

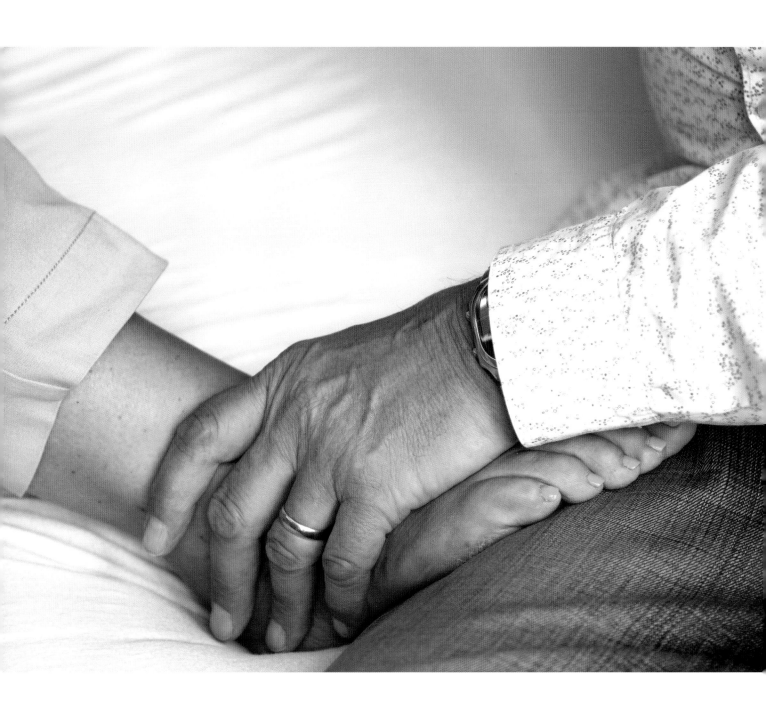

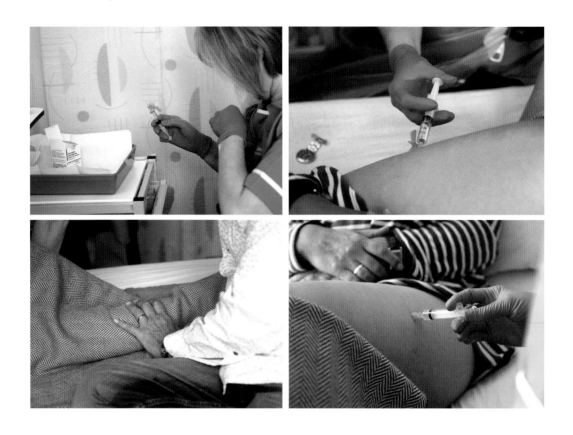

3 January 2015

So there we are. It is all done. Yesterday was my 43rd visit to hospital for the 9th and final Herceptin jab. I should have been jubilant. Instead I felt sad for all the other patients whose treatment is still ongoing.

Back home the first letter I opened was from the hospital asking me to come for a mammogram in three weeks. What? Is this Groundhog Day? While I am grateful for the experience and insight this journey has given me, I certainly would not want to face it again.

I have taken to my bed today. My kidneys ache and I am tired. We finally moved in to Manor Farm House just before Christmas. Oh to be reunited with our big sleigh bed that spent my entire treatment time in storage. And oh the new view from it. We look for miles across rolling Dorset countryside. It is wonderful. That in itself is a blessing.

The scales have also appeared from storage. I had to face them this morning. I am half a stone heavier than the heaviest I have ever been. Crikey. It is now time to address this. I like the latest fad for the alkaline diet. In that an acidic body gets cancer, this seems to be a fad that I should follow. I have ordered two books .

But I have to do more than alkalise my body. Meditation has to become a regular practice. I need to up my yoga and exercise routines. But above all I need to focus on my goals and my dreams.

Reconstruction

19 March 2015

" It is the light at the end of the tunnel.
More than that, it is a wonderful gift."

19 March 2015

Back at the hospital and delighted to be here for once as I'm waiting to meet Mr Masood - a plastic surgeon...

OK, so one nipple is 4cm lower than the other. It felt like I was being measured for a suit. It has been agreed that not only will they reduce the left down in size to match the right, but that they will reduce them both, thus hiding evidence of the lumpectomy.

It is the light at the end of the tunnel. More than that, it is a wonderful gift. Though Mr Masood was not amused when I cheekily asked for a bit of liposuction at the same time. The answer was a flat 'No'.

28 April 2015

Johnnie burst into tears when I lifted my surgical gown. "What's wrong?"

"You've got the tits of a 21 year old... It's amazing."

I only came out of surgery five hours ago so they are covered in dressings (with heart shaped nipple flaps). But from what I can judge they look incredibly pert, neat and SMALL. What a transformation. H to a C. Mercy me.

Not only are they smaller (and the same size) the scar and lump in the right breast has been completely removed. It is just incredible.

There's no mirror in here so I get Johnnie to take a photo on my phone so I can better gauge their size. Holly Moses. I am totally transformed. (By the end of the day this photo has been sent to at least five people.)

Happily I'm not too sore. I have a drain at the side of each breast to collect the blood but that is a minor inconvenience.

I am in my own room – overlooking fields. I have to pinch myself I feel so lucky. A couple of days in here being looked after will suit me just fine.

7 May 2015

A big day. The country is electing its future leader and the my new 'puppies' are being revealed to me when the dressing is removed. I have been elated all week. People telling me I look 3 stone lighter and feeling like a totally new woman. It is the most liberating thing that has ever happened to me. I feel normal now, not a freak.

But my elation was shattered when I saw them. Dear God – the stitches. I look like Frankenstein's bride. That shock and the sheer effort of going to the hospital and then to vote sent me in to decline. I slept all afternoon.

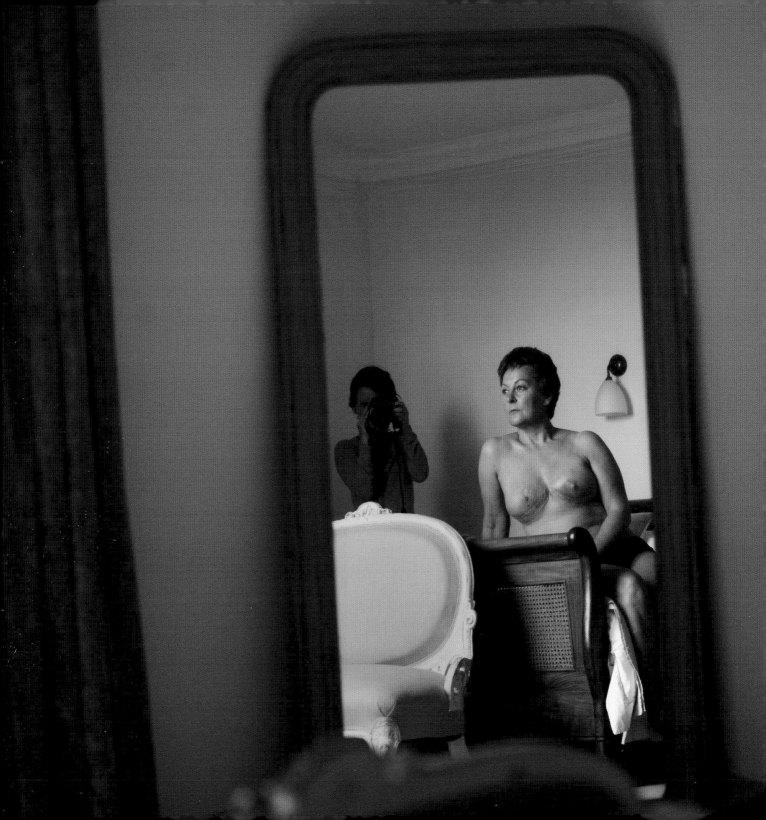

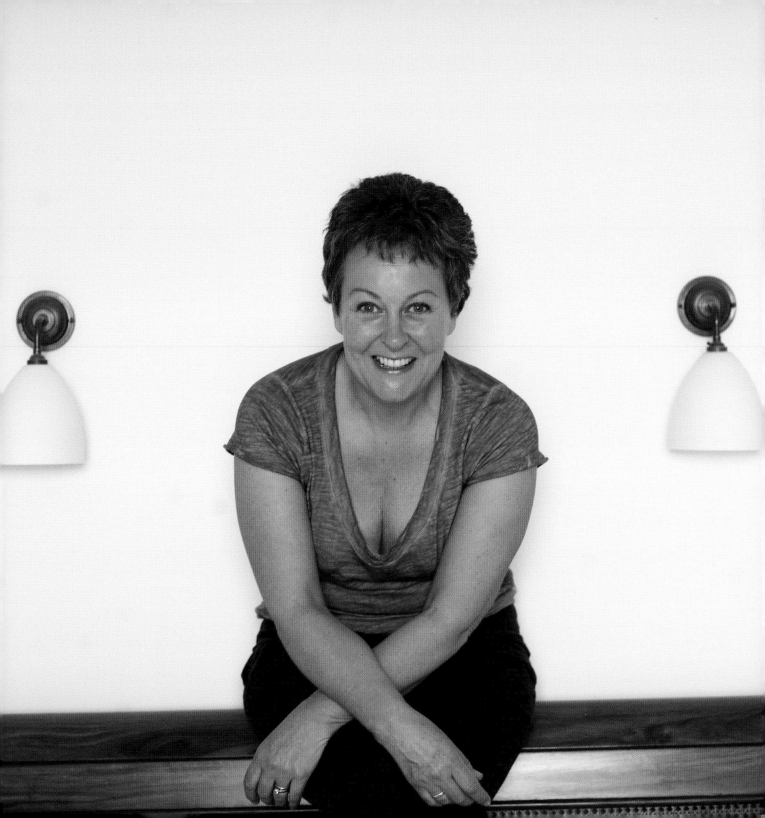

14 May 2015

Today the final dressing was removed. I also saw Mr Masood. He was pleased with his handy work but warned they would take several months to settle down. "Don't buy expensive bras yet." Was that aimed at Johnnie or me? He also reported that the breast tissue removed tested negative for any more cancerous cells. I knew it would, but it's pretty fantastic to have my instinct confirmed.

I tried to thank him, to tell him how amazing it is what he has done for me. But he's a humble man and was not open to praise. When I think about it, every nurse and doctor has been the same. They do their jobs well because they take pride in them. I've not met one ego. And people knock the NHS. I think it is incredible.

As Johnnie and I walked down the corridor I thought, well that's it. The journey is over. Now I really can get on with my life.

And the fact is that it will be a very different life. A lot has changed for me in the past eighteen months. Not just my body – although having smaller breasts is extremely profound. My priorities have shifted. I was an out and out 'doer'. I was spinning around, always frantic, yet I wasn't actually achieving anything fulfilling for me. Now my focus is on getting rid of the unnecessary. I need less in my life, not more. I need time and space. Not stress and fatigue. I am moving to a place where I want to 'be' rather than 'do'. And now I have an excuse to say, 'No'.

The things that I do sit with – in particular my writing – will have space to breath, to grow, to manifest. It is so often quoted that 'less is more'. I truly believe that is the case. I'm not sure I would have learnt that without the past eighteen months.

Funny how life works out.

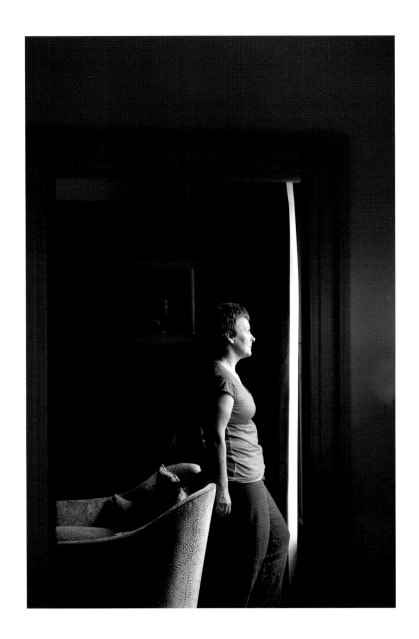

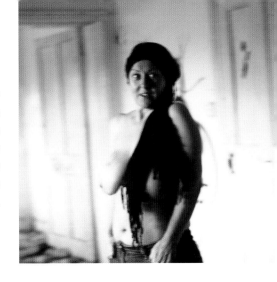

Acknowledgments

I would like to thank Johnnie for being my tireless carer; the Staff of Salisbury District Hospital especially surgeons Vicky Brown and Mr Masood, Dr Claire Crowley and the nurses on the Pembroke Suite; the radiotherapy team at Poole Hospital; my parents; friends who walked the dog and brought us meals; my alternative support crew - Carole Saunders, Salil the needle, Sarah Fairy, Tony Monkcom; Carly Cook and Susan d'Arcy for editorial guidance and finally Bella West for joining me at every stage of this unplanned journey with her camera, great eye and humour.

Tiggy Walker
July 2015

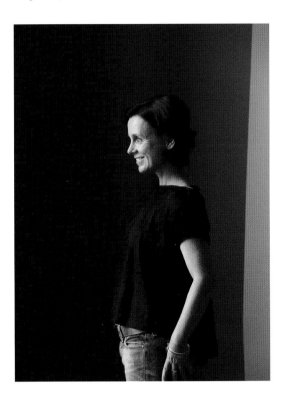

Bella West has been at the forefront of photographic portraiture for 20 years. In that time, she has been awarded for her outstanding work not only within the portrait field but through her sensitive imagery, documentuary stills and childrens fashion. Her versatility and skill using available light, coupled with a sensitive energy, gives her work individuality and commercial impact, allowing her to work in variable genres within the fashion & editorial fields.

Her vivid style of contemporary classical portraiture, yet with a colourful flare for storytelling, enables her to produce work for her clients which goes beyond the norm, utilising location, texture and graphic.

A passionate lecturer and judge, Bella currently holds a Fellowhship and sits on the BIPP Board of Directors. She has two published works to date.

www.bellawest.co.uk

©Bella West 2015

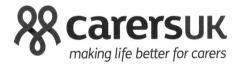

Royalties from this book are being donated to Carers UK.
Tiggy and Johnnie Walker are Patrons of the 50th Anniversary Appeal.
Charity No. 246329
www.carersuk.org

Tiggys email arrived on 17th January 2014 and despite my own heavy heart at the news, really my first thoughts were of admiration at her boldness to consider this project so early on in her diagnosis, It would take strength to be offering herself to me in this way. Had she any idea how vulnerable she could feel? How exposed she may potentially be?

I'm sure we all think hard about what we can do in a practical sense when we hear news like this. Sympathise of course, in an emotional sense, but on a practical level we want to help, it's natural. Whether this be driving to appointments, soup making, dog walking or just someone to scream at. Being conscioius of how life will change for those concerened, how can we help with that if at all?

Tiggys request for photographs, portraits of her to be taken in exposed state, was a nod to her optimistic mechanism maybe to offer a distraction and most certainly a goal. Tiggy and I were familiar with each other purely through having mutual friends, she wasn't asking this from a close friend, so it was a professional commission on my part which removed the emotional attachment.

Photography is about giving. A picture, every photograph ever taken, or to be taken, is unique, a one off. No technology can ever supersede that. A moment in photograph form, is something you can give which noone else will have, it's two fingers to the power of money or status. It's not always obvious that photography is something we give, it can be seen as being gratuitous just through not having clarity in the message or by just leaving the viewer asking 'why?' or indeed the manner in which it was taken. My short spell in Rwanda clarified to me the power that photography has to tell a story, to educate and to an extent, to assist with the healing through a visual portrayal of reality that may offer some comfort. This project could potentially reach out to millions of people.

To take this project on, took me all of the time to make a cuppa to consider - engaging in personal projects is a fundamental part of my creative and personal growth. By placing myself in situations which are uncomfortable & challenging on a personal and professional level, and making me consider the approach that both tells the story but without sensationalising a situation. It's not always about taking the most obvious and pushing for something that perhaps isn't there, more about allowing the story to tell itself.

So I'd like to explain what this project isn't.

The images I have taken of Tiggy are not to show one single element of her journey. It's not designed to make her look brave or not scared, nor to make her look beautiful. Or not. It goes deeper than being just brave and it is a representation of honesty and a very real portrayal of her treatment on a physical and emotional level. Tiggy's tenacity offered me creative freedom from the outset and anything I offered her, she accepted. I could have just made pictures which made her look beautiful but then we wouldn't have the story we have here.

I have documented Tiggy for a year in order to perhaps answer some questions for those that are about to venture into the terrifying world of cancer. It seems to me, despite support networks, the immense work of the NHS and their staff, that this is still a personal and often isolated battle for both patient and carer.. The images, that sit alongside Tiggys diary writing aims to invite the reader into her world of initial acceptance, her strength of charachter, her humour and pure resilience to be beaten down.

This has been a journey, unplanned, for all of us.

Bella West
2015